PTSD AND THE POLITICS OF TRAUMA IN ISRAEL

A Nation on the Couch

Post-traumatic stress disorder, or PTSD, has long been understood as a mental trauma that affects the individual. However, what role do families, health experts, and the national community at large play in interpreting and responding to this individualized trauma?

In *PTSD and the Politics of Trauma in Israel*, Keren Friedman-Peleg sheds light on a new way of speaking about mental vulnerability and national belonging in contemporary Israel. Based on ethnographic fieldwork conducted at the Israel Center for Victims of Terror and War and the Israel Trauma Coalition between 2004 and 2009, Friedman-Peleg's rich ethnographic study challenges the traditional and limited definitions of trauma. In doing so, she exposes how these clinical definitions have been transformed into new categories of identity, thereby raising new dynamics of power, as well as new forms of dialogue.

KEREN FRIEDMAN-PELEG is a senior lecturer at the School of Behavioral Sciences and the Head of the President's Program for Excellence at the College of Management – Academic Studies in Israel.

PTSD and the Politics of Trauma in Israel

A Nation on the Couch

KEREN FRIEDMAN-PELEG

UNIVERSITY OF TORONTO PRESS
Toronto Buffalo London

© University of Toronto Press 2017
Toronto Buffalo London
www.utppublishing.com
Printed in the U.S.A.

First edition published by The Hebrew University Magnes Press,
Jerusalem, 2014: העם על הספה: הפוליטיקה של הטראומה בישראל, קרן פרידמן-פלג

ISBN 978-1-4426-5051-0 (cloth)   ISBN 978-1-4426-2931-8 (paper)

 Printed on acid-free, 100% post-consumer recycled paper with
vegetable-based inks.

Library and Archives Canada Cataloguing in Publication

Friedman-Peleg, Keren, 1975–
[ha-`Am `al ha-sapah. English]
PTSD and the politics of trauma in Israel : a nation on the couch / Keren
Friedman-Peleg.

First edition published by The Hebrew University Magnes Press, Jerusalem,
2014 under title: ha-`Am `al ha-sapah : ha-poli‚ti‚kah shel ha-‚tra`umah
be-Yi´sra`el.

Includes bibliographical references and index.
ISBN 978-1-4426-5051-0 (cloth). – ISBN 978-1-4426-2931-8 (paper)

1. Post-traumatic stress disorder – Israel.   2. Soldiers – Israel – Psychological
aspects.   3. Traumatic shock – Israel – Case studies.   I. Title.   II. Title:
ha-`Am `al ha-sapah. English

RC552.P67F7613 2017   616.85'21   C2016-905114-5

University of Toronto Press acknowledges the financial assistance to its
publishing program of the Canada Council for the Arts and the Ontario Arts
Council, an agency of the Government of Ontario.

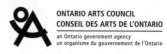

To my mother, Ahuva
(who taught me the power of words in Hebrew),

To my father, Eitan
(who taught me the power of words in English),

And for both of them:
For prayers they have made, and for great loves –
To daily life, to work, to Israel, to the kibbutz,
to one another, and for us

Contents

Acknowledgments

Many days and long nights have come together to make the publishing of this book not only a possible mission but also a fruitful journey, full of moments of joy and even a few, crucial epiphanies.

First, I would like to thank the supervisors of my PhD dissertation: Professors Yoram Bilu and Moshe Shokeid. To Yoram I owe a deep thank-you for the hand he agreed to hold at just the right moment when it seemed that anthropology and psychology were refusing to be investigated together, and for helping me to see the enormous potential of blending individual matters with collective concerns. Yoram's supervision was a very constructive journey we took together behind the secret confines of the clinic, when theoretical lenses and empirical findings were mixed with raising children – my daughters and his grandchildren. Moshe is the first and my most important teacher of anthropology. During the hot summer of 1996, a few months after the political murder of Prime Minister Yitzhak Rabin, he opened the door for me and showed me a world where interacting with other human beings and facing their fears, wishes, dreams, and loves (while facing your own fears, wishes, dreams, and loves) was the most important aspect of a good ethnography.

While being closely engaged with the mental vulnerability of individuals, families, and communities inside Israel, there have been anthropologists from abroad who have become outstanding teachers for me. Allan Young is the first. Reading his seminal work, *The Harmony of Illusion: Inventing Post-Traumatic Stress Disorder* (published by Princeton University Press in 1995), and then meeting with Allan himself were among the most meaningful and stimulating experiences I had during my ethnographic research about security-related PTSD in Israel. Allan's kind willingness to become a close mentor of mine was, and still is, crucial to my ability to publish my local ethnography outside the borders of Israel. Being aware of Allan's powerful research about the diagnostic category of PTSD became a gateway into the works of other anthropologists who provide ongoing inspiration to my investigation into the global-local interplay surrounding the professional therapy of trauma. Given this growing field in psychological and medical anthropology, there are certainly too many to be mentioned, but nonetheless I'd like to extend my great appreciation and thanks to five important figures in this field: Didier Fassin, Erica James, Laurence Kirmayer, Michael Lambek, and Tanya Luhrmann.

The Department of Sociology and Anthropology at Tel Aviv University was my first home after I left my parents' home on the kibbutz. I would like to thank all the department's teachers to whom I listened and who were willing to listen me; whose texts I read and who were willing to read mine, especially Ofra Goldstein-Gidoni, Hanna Herzog, Adriana Kemp, Danny Rabinowitz, Ronen Shamir, and Yehuda Shenhav. I owe a special thanks to Haim Hazan for providing miles of wisdom and sensitivity between Van Leer Jerusalem Institute and Tel Aviv, and to Nissim Mizrachi who taught me about anthropological sociology, and sociological anthropology, and especially for ongoing mentoring. A deep thanks also to Tamar El-Or for the kibbutz, the city, and the words in-between; and to Yehuda Goodman, Carol Kidron, Amalia Sa'ar, and Zahava Solomon for very constructive comments and feedback along the way.

The College of Management–Academic Studies is my second and contemporary academic home. I would like to thank the College's president, Asher Tishler, the head of the board of directors, Ron Gutler, and the following key figures at the College: Rani Jaconi, Carmela Jacobi-Valk, Mylli Ellis, Yoram Eden, Michal Gilboa, Esti Matza-Rom, Gali Sarogati, Rafi Gamish, and Liat Hazani. Within the college, the School of Behavioral Sciences is my professional anchor. I would like to thank my former dean, Dalia Mor, and the current one, Rachel Pasternak, and my colleagues: Shula Ben-Ari, Gadi Ben-Ezer, Anat Guy, Bat Katzman, Oleg Komlik, and Avi Shnieder. A special thanks to Limor Chen, my incredible teaching assistant who is a brilliant young scholar in her own right. I would also like to thank my students from the School of Behavioral Sciences and from the President's Program for Excellence for their willingness to join me, every week, one semester after another, to journey into the world of trauma and resilience, and actually into the life of all of us. I love you all very much.

Between January and May 2016, I had the great honour of being a fellow at the Katz Center for Advanced Judaic Studies at the University of Pennsylvania. As a native Israeli, and as an anthropologist who deals with trauma in the contemporary context of Israel, the opportunity to take part in an ongoing dialogue about Judaism and Jews, while being exposed to the high professional standards of the Center, has had no less than a transformative meaning for me. The power of being a fellow at the Katz Center was connected to the strict academic requirements (i.e., to elaborate my research skills thanks to weekly seminars and daily encounters with scholars from different fields) and to the opportunity of being involved in an ongoing dialogue with the broader Jewish and non-Jewish community of Philadelphia and beyond. I would like to express my deep gratitude to Tom Katz, whose father's pioneering way of thinking gave the community at the Center a chance to thrive, and to Steven Weitzman, the Center's director, for his so kind and stimulating leadership. It is a great pleasure to extend my thanks to all the fellows who were at the Center during the 2015–16 academic year, and especially to John Efron, Galit Hasan-Rokem, Martin Kavka, Arthur Kiron, Lital Levi, Rachel Werczberger, and Rakefet Zalashik.

The University of Toronto Press was the first publisher I approached when I decided to take the first step towards the publication of my ethnography. I was fortunate enough to receive an answer of "Yes." It has been a very constructive journey, from the first version I submitted to the Press to the final manuscript. I would like to extend my deep thanks to my editors: Eric Carlson who began this journey with me, and Stephen Shapiro who ended it. Both Eric and Stephen were kind and sharp readers, and very professional editors. I also found these high standards in Lisa Jemison, assistant managing editor, and in the work of freelance editor Beth McAuley. Nonetheless, it is worth mentioning that all this wonderful work by UTP's editorial staff would not be possible without the initial process of translating and editing my dissertation from Hebrew to English. I would like to send my appreciation to the Israeli editors with whom I worked: Frances Zetland, Ruvik Danieli, and especially Amy Fields, who worked hard, very hard, on the final version of the manuscript.

To the trauma experts from NATAL (the Israel Trauma Center for Victims of Terror and War) and ITC (the Israel Trauma Coalition), the two Israeli NGOs that are the centre of my ethnographic research, I owe a big thanks for their willingness to make room for an anthropologist in their aid agencies, and for their unusual openness to expose their daily work to an external gaze. During my long hours at NATAL, Judith Yovel-Recanati, Orly Gal, Avi Bleich, Itamar Barnea, Sa'ar Uzieli, and Sigal Haimov were kind enough to allow me to be a professional like them, as well as a patient like all the women, men, and families they have met with. A big thanks to Talia Levanon, the ITC's CEO, whose outstanding courage and braveness paved the way for me into the ITC's council meetings. Many thanks to the psychiatrists and psychologists from all the NGOs who joined together in this innovative collaboration, and especially to the ones from MASHABIM ICSPC (the Community Stress and Prevention Center), ICMC (Israel Crisis Management Center, or SELAH in Hebrew), AMCHA (after the code word that helped survivors identify fellow Jews during the Holocaust), the Psycho-trauma Center in Jerusalem, and ERAN (Emotional First Aid).

While bringing this manuscript into its last version, I received grants from the Research Authority at the College of Management–Academic Studies and from the School of Behavioral Sciences at the College. Conducting a prolonged, multi-sited ethnography like mine could only be possible thanks to the kind and stable financial support I have received over the years from the Pollak Foundation Scholarship, Tel Aviv University (2004–8), from the Rector's Scholarship for Excellent Students, Tel Aviv University (2004–8), and from Saymon Reispous Foundation, Tel Aviv University (2007). I also received invaluable financial support from the Ginsburg Foundation during my postdoctoral fellowship at the Department of Sociology and Anthropology at the Hebrew University of Jerusalem (2008–9), and during my postdoctoral fellowship at the Department of Medical Education at the Sackler Medical School of Tel Aviv University (2010–11). I am deeply grateful.

Finally, I want to close by telling one of the mythological stories that makes the rounds between the generations of my family. It describes how, at the end of the 1970s, my parents, who were living on a kibbutz, were invited to meet one of the most famous and influential dancers in Israel, whom I will call Ms. Levin. The reason for the invitation was that my older sister's great qualities as a dancer had caught Ms. Levin's eye. She came to the meeting with an unusual offer for my parents: she invited them to send my sister abroad so that she could become part of a professional ensemble of dancers in New York City. It almost goes without saying, yet it is worth mentioning, that at that time Israel in general, and our small kibbutz in particular, seemed to be very, very far from New York City, much more than today. Both of my parents – my father who was born in Tel Aviv to a father who came to Israel from Germany and to a mother who was of Yameni origin, and my mother who was born in Jerusalem to Jewish immigrants from Iraq and Syria – had never had a chance to visit New York City or to take their children for such a visit. "Dad, you know him," my mum likes to say. "He heard the name New York and immediately became enthusiastic." "Well, Ahu," my mum recalled he said to her (he used to shorten her first name, Ahuva, as a sign of love), "just think about it, she will be an international!" "Friedman," my mum replied (she used to call him by our last name, Friedman, instead of his first name, Eitan, as a sign of love), "instead of sending her so far from home, why don't you become an international?!"

In the end, my sister didn't move to NYC, and she regrets it to this day. Actually, none of us has become an "international." Similar to our parents, we are very attached to Israel, and to the day-to-day, sometimes painful, life here. Yet I am guessing that by publishing this book, in English, to an audience outside of Israel, I will find my own way of dancing between here and there, between locality and internationality, between the kibbutz and all those New York places. I dedicate this dance to the Friedman family – to my parents, my brother and two sisters, their spouses, children, and grandchildren, and to my own, lovely family: my beloved spouse, Idan, and our two one-of-a kind daughters, Noga and Mika.

Finally, one last comment: during the long months of working on this manuscript, I had contradictory thoughts regarding the most appropriate way to present the main figures from NATAL and ITC throughout the chapters of the book. On the one hand, instead of pseudonyms I prefer open descriptions, full names, and titles. On the other hand, the complexity of the therapeutic work and the processes of marketing and fundraising raised concerns about compromising the privacy of the NATAL and ITC experts. Eventually, I chose the middle path. I present the two organizations by their full names, as well as the main philanthropic forces behind them. Regarding the internal discussions of NATAL, I refer to all the senior experts and administrators, with their consent, by their full names and professional titles. However, I refer to the ITC senior members and donors with pseudonyms, and I have obscured their personal and professional titles. The identity of anyone who received aid was kept fully confidential.

PTSD AND THE POLITICS OF TRAUMA IN ISRAEL

A Nation on the Couch

Introduction

Beyond the Secret Confines of the Clinic: An Ethnographic Journey Tracing the Politics of Trauma in Israel

The ethnographic journey of this book began one morning in August 2006 at the mayor's office in Sderot, a town in Israel's southern periphery. Ever since the town's residents were first exposed to Qassam rocket fire from the Gaza Strip in April 2001, this office had seen countless meetings and visits. Nevertheless, on that morning, the gathering in the mayor's office was exceptional. The municipality spokesperson stood tensely facing clinical psychologists and psychiatrists from local non-governmental organizations (NGOs) based in the centre of the country, along with representatives from the United Jewish Agency-Federation of New York (UJA-Federation). These Jewish-American donors were the financial backers of an aid program operated by the therapists in Sderot for the purpose of treating many of the town's residents who had developed post-traumatic symptoms in the wake of repeated rocket fire. Together with the local trauma experts, the donors had come to the town for a weeklong solidarity visit to take a closer look at the aid program. A busy itinerary was planned for the UJA-Federation's representatives in Sderot, but the first stop was the mayor's office, and the first speaker was the municipality spokesperson. The attendees gathered around the long table, some sitting, but most standing, listening attentively to the spokesperson as he began the meeting:

> Good morning everyone, and welcome to Sderot. It is a great honour for us to host you here this morning ... Until April 2001, no one even imagined that Qassam rockets or any rockets at all would reach Sderot ... There is a lot of fear, a lot of trauma, a lot wounded physically, and there are thousands wounded emotionally ... The assistance has been much appreciated, but it isn't enough. (24 August 2006, Field Notes)

At this slightly awkward moment, as the spokesperson asked for additional financial aid from the Jewish-American donors right at the beginning of their visit, a senior clinical psychologist, who was working at one of the NGOs that was leading the aid program in Sderot, interrupted him. The psychologist stopped the spokesperson in order to translate his opening remarks from Hebrew to English so the UJA-Federation representatives could easily understand him. Then he turned to the municipality spokesperson and told him, "Make it snappy, you've only got five minutes."

SPOKESPERSON (in surprise): Five minutes? But you told me I could speak for ten minutes!

PSYCHOLOGIST: That's right, but you don't speak English, and the translation takes time. That leaves us only five minutes.

SPOKESPERSON (angrily): You don't want me to talk? You're insulting me … If you're in a hurry – go! You've all come here to hear us! … All the assistance that's been given to Sderot is welcome, but all of you have got to understand that an entire city is in trauma! (24 August 2006, Field Notes)

The Sderot spokesperson's remarks illustrate how the expression of gratitude has become wrapped up in descriptions of trauma. These remarks, from someone who was not a mental health expert but rather involved with the media, demonstrate how, over the past two decades, security-based trauma has found its way into the public discourse in Israel. Contrary to the suffering that results from natural disasters or socio-economic causes, when I use security-based trauma in Israel I am referring to the emotional experience of fear, anxiety, helplessness, and other related emotions caused by the geopolitical conflict between Israel, the Palestinians, and the neighbouring Arab states. The clinical construct of trauma, which has enjoyed periods of discovery as well as times of marginality in Western mental health discourse (Herman, 1992; Kutchins and Kirk, 1997; Young, 1995), has penetrated the fabric of daily life in Israel. Mental trauma has become not just an emotional experience characterizing the private world of many Israeli citizens but also a phenomenon whose very existence is marked and talked about in order to garner recognition and aid.

At the same time, the outbursts accompanying this new talk about trauma points to the tense dynamic that has developed around this diagnostic. The description of the mental distress was delivered in Hebrew by the spokesperson from a town under attack, a Jew whose North African ("Mizrachi") origin was revealed in his speech. Then, a local clinical psychologist of upper-middle-class Eastern European ("Ashkenazi") origin interrupted the spokesperson to translate the information into English for Jewish-American donors. Next, when further interrupted by a new request to hurry up and be brief, the spokesperson expressed anger and humiliation. The social dynamic around the mental trauma, therefore, took place among different social players from various institutions and from diverse political perspectives, prompting a mini power struggle: Who has the right to speak on behalf of those experiencing mental trauma? In which language? For how long? Five minutes? Ten? And to what purpose?

The above ethnographic description provides the starting point from which I embarked on a journey to examine how the mental condition of trauma has been defined not only as an individual experience but also as an emotional one that an entire national community needs to interpret and respond to. What happens when an Israeli husband has been diagnosed with PTSD as a result of his military service? What is a wife's role regarding commitment, love, and intimacy? And what if she herself has been diagnosed with "secondary trauma"? When Israeli soldiers have had their masculine identity threatened by experiences of fear and helplessness in the battlefield during the Second Lebanon War or a military operation in Gaza Strip, how can they come to terms with it? When urban communities in the south and north of Israel are subjected to rocket fire, how can these populations be stabilized? And what goes on when they meet mental health experts who offer them therapeutic tools? When marketing advisers need to "sell" traumatic experiences inside and outside the borders of Israel for the sake of raising public awareness (and money), how should this be accomplished? When Jewish-American donors feel obligated to help and support, how do they perceive their role? What happens when the mental health experts themselves – psychiatrists, clinical psychologists, psychotherapists, and social workers – become involved in an ongoing negotiation over the meaning and treatment of PTSD and trauma under the current security circumstances in Israel?

From the outset, this journey has understood trauma as a "text": something that "depends upon yet transcends both performance and audience, reader and text, the material object and a reflective, sensuous response" (Good, 1994: 167). Rather than keeping trauma behind the closed doors of the clinic, assuming it to be a natural and universal emotional condition, I trace the myriad connections between the painful experiences of trauma, core national values, and organizational commitments.

I am doing so based on the fieldwork I conducted from 2004 to 2009 at two NGOs: NATAL (Israel Center for Victims of Terror and War, established in 1998) and the umbrella organization, ITC (Israel Trauma Coalition, established three years later in 2001; NATAL was among the first NGOs invited to join ITC). My work focuses on trauma and post-trauma management in relation to three landmark events in the Arab–Israeli conflict: (1) the Second Intifada of October 2000, (2) the Disengagement Plan of August 2005, and (3) the Second Lebanon War of July 2006.

I conducted participatory observations at a variety of settings where clinical psychologists and psychiatrists from NATAL and ITC conducted therapeutic work. I attended the meetings of clinical psychologists and documented their professional debates about how to treat a soldier who had been held captive by Syrians or Egyptians, or a soldier who had mistakenly shot to death a comrade-in-arms during combat activity. I documented ITC council meetings where the local therapists considered how to present the anguish of Israeli border residents to the Jewish-American donors from New York. I observed the process of establishing "haven rooms" in Sderot elementary schools during the spring and summer of 2006. A few months prior to that, I observed meetings with groups of soldiers who had served during the Second Intifada and refused to accept mental aid. I attended "empathy practice sessions" that were held for religious Jewish mentors who lived in Jewish settlements in the Gaza Strip just before the Disengagement Plan in the summer months of 2005, and a seminar for bereaved Druze parents held that same summer. In September 2005, I witnessed an intensive day of filming for a movie that one of the NGOs was producing. This multi-sited ethnography is the foundation of this book, and each setting that I examined allowed me to view the professional approach towards trauma from another angle.

However, the nature of this ethnographic quest that goes beyond the clinical scope of trauma carried within it an inherent challenge. Like other experts in modern society, those involved in providing therapeutic aid usually perceive themselves, and are so perceived by the public, as being highly autonomous. That autonomy extends to having the authority to determine who may and may not pass through the gates of the professional community, and to whom and how they, as experts, should provide aid (Gieryn, 1999). The common assumption is that empirical evidence and scientific tools are the basis for therapeutic aid, and thus, the experts applying it are protected from any limitations of moral judgment or social prejudices. It is, at least partly, on this basis that the experts have drawn a clear line between them and the lay people, delineating who did and did not belong to the professional community (Murphy, 1988). Thus, for an outsider, to gaze upon the daily activities of this exclusive community was by no means an easy task.

Nevertheless, my journey into the secret confines of the clinic and beyond was made possible by the personal relationships I gradually developed with the trauma experts from NATAL and ITC. All the while, I remained highly aware of the differences that might exist between us, that we held different professional positions – I was an anthropologist, they were mental health experts – and as such we might have different perspectives (Shokeid, 1997) on "what is at stake" when dealing with security-based trauma. In March 2004, I met Gali Dagan who was then in charge of NATAL's public relations. Dagan was a bit sceptical about the actual possibility of conducting anthropological research at NATAL, but allowed me to present the idea to Dr. Itamar Barnea, the NGO's chief psychologist. After perusing my curriculum vitae and an abstract of my dissertation, the NATAL steering committee invited me to a meeting. Besides Barnea, all the heads of the NGO's professional teams and the committee chair, Professor Avi Bleich, attended the meeting. The anthropological viewpoint turned out to be of intriguing promise to those who had spent most of their professional lives dealing with quantitative research and to an NGO that is highly aware of how others perceive its activities (Shamir, 2008; Silber, 2008). I offered them what people are often lacking and what lies at the heart of anthropological research: time – my time, together with documentation and interpretation. The heads of the teams promised me their (almost) full cooperation, and they delivered.

At the start of the fieldwork, I conducted semi-structured, in-depth interviews with NATAL therapists, members of the marketing team, and administrators. More than thirty interviews facilitated the development of mutual trust and laid the groundwork for the next stage of the study: participant observation. For a period of five years, I was present at diverse settings where clinical psychologists and therapists conducted therapeutic work. These included situations such as psycho-social interventions among various groups of Israeli residents and training processes among local caregivers. In addition, I documented what took place at different settings where discussions and debates transpired regarding the therapeutic work, such as meetings of the NGO's steering committee or meetings of the professional teams. However, the door to the clinic, and within it the iconic couch we identify with therapy, remained shut to me. Time would pass until I accessed the room and discovered that the couch had been transformed. Behind those doors, the couch often took the form of folding chairs, long benches, or ragged mats upon which various social players from diverse social locations and with a variety of political interests debated the treatment of trauma.

I arrived at ITC pursuant to my fieldwork at NATAL. Together with other NGOs, NATAL was among the first to be invited to join ITC upon its establishment, a year after the outbreak of the Second Intifada. The aim of the invitation was to found a "super-NGO," that is, a network of organizations that would provide Israel's citizens with coordinated, diverse, and long-term therapeutic aid. In hindsight, the willingness of ITC administrators to pave my way into the council meetings appears to have stemmed from coincidence. Michal Amitai-Tehori, then director general of NATAL, referred me to ITC, whose senior staff saw this as a sign of NATAL's acceptance of their authority. However, it was unclear to them whether I represented NATAL or myself. Later, when ITC's senior staff understood the situation more clearly, I had already laid the foundation for the ethnographic research, making it easier to continue. At the first ITC council meeting, which I attended in August 2005, I introduced myself and presented the anthropological perspective on security-based trauma that I wanted to pursue. Quite surprisingly, during the first few months, I was asked to repeat this explanation at almost every council meeting. This was contrary to NATAL, where the process of my entry into the organization was slow and gradual, and eventually I became completely immersed in what transpired there. At ITC, I spent an entire year entering and exiting the field, before I managed to establish my presence. After almost a year of participant observations at the council meetings, I volunteered to record meeting protocols. This tactic helped me normalize my presence at the council meetings, even after a new secretary joined and took over this task.

Using the rich findings I collected from five years of close observation of the professional work of NATAL and ITC, I undertook a critical analysis of how the mental conditions of security-based trauma have been managed in Israel, but one which remained alert and sensitive to the complexities involved in providing and receiving mental aid. In shaping this as the object of my analysis, I found myself in an interesting dialogue with critical theories of social sciences and cultural studies that often introduce the appearance of the therapeutic discourse as a new, sophisticated, and elusive form of power. Presenting the "soul" as the main site for observation, classification, and categorization, even if based on soft tools such as conversations with an expert, these theories claim that psychology and psychiatry are anything but another way to gain social control over the individual. However, in contrast to this tendency to distinguish categorically between those who have the knowledge and the power to control and subordinate those who do not,[1] I chose to remain aware of the social circumstances under which the therapeutic interventions took place. The complexity of dealing with trauma under the particular security circumstances of Israel demanded that I not assume in advance the existence of categorical relationships between the aid providers, as carriers of highly legitimate scientific knowledge, and the receivers, as those who lack knowledge. Instead, I conducted my ethnographic research based on the assumptions that the experts were social players operating under some social limitations while being sensitive to the flexibility and creativity they expressed and, finally, while considering how the clinical construct of trauma has touched various sociopolitical groups while its definition and effects have been debated in multiple venues.

Five years of fieldwork at NATAL and ITC, therefore, revealed how far the professional approach towards security-based trauma is from

---

1 This position is mainly identified with the post-structuralist theory of French philosopher Michel Foucault. Foucault characterized modern society as constituting a disciplinary system of knowledge and power, the purpose of which is to make the modern individual a rational subject and decent citizen. Therapeutic knowledge was one of the foci on which Foucault based his argument. Just as a priest promises believers redemption and thus establishes his/her authority with them, so too does therapeutic knowledge build its authority. In the name of the claim to "truth," the various manifestations of this power – the hospitals, prisons, and schools – link the individual with his/her identity and impose a variety of disciplinary practices on the subject (Foucault, 1973). For an extended sociopolitical analysis within this theoretical framework, see Rose (1998).

being evidenced-based. I shed light on how closely this clinical construct has intertwined with sociopolitical issues of class and ethnic differences as well as those of national belonging. Eventually, this blend of individual's symptoms of psychopathology with sociocultural markers from daily life in Israel evoked a metamorphosis in the local meaning of trauma, while redefining the raison d'être of both the aid providers and aid receivers.

Trauma and the Anthropological Discourse:
The Interplay between Globalization and Localization

The word "trauma" was not a word used in common English when it was in the hands of surgeons treating mutilated soldiers; it was one of those fancy words that lay people didn't use, and often did not even understand. But now, "traumatic experience" and all the other uses of trauma are standard English words.
        –Ian Hacking, "Memory Science, Memory Politics" (1996: 75)

This definition by philosopher Ian Hacking fittingly describes the dynamic history of trauma within Western mental health discourse. During the last century, the professional approach towards life-threatening events has alternated between periods of intense clinical inquiry and periods of complete marginality (Herman, 1992; Kutchins and Kirk, 1997). However, the most dramatic shift in the way we understand trauma seems to have occurred with the disorder's institutionalization in the DSM-III (1980). The work of various key figures within psychiatry were undoubtedly responsible for this change, especially the strong Vietnam veterans' lobby. In his pioneering book, *The Harmony of Illusions: Inventing Posttraumatic Stress Disorder* (1995), medical anthropologist Allan Young argued that the major motivation for the publication of the disorder was not scientific-empirical but rather political. Based on historical and ethnographic research, Young shows that the generally accepted view of post-traumatic stress disorder (PTSD), and of the traumatic memory that underlies it, is inaccurate. The disorder, he claims, is not timeless nor does it represent a singular substantial entity: "Rather, it is glued together by the practices, technologies, and the narratives with which it is diagnosed, studied, treated, and represented by the various interests, institutions, and moral arguments that mobilize these efforts and resources" (Young, 1995: 5).

After PTSD was institutionalized in the DSM-III and following Young's foundational research, the anthropological study of the disorder has primarily dealt with the issue of global-local interplay surrounding the treatment of the disorder and how local politics has figured into this diagnostic category. This ethnographic focus has produced two major theoretical directions. While the first direction focuses on how local forms of suffering have been translated into one, Western-oriented clinical concept, the second explores the specific cultural meaning that the clinical concept of trauma has absorbed in different local sites. The first body of anthropological literature emphasizes how the DSM-III classification both medicalized and depoliticized the experiences of mental vulnerability and suffering. Anthropologists have shown how mental experts treated the victims as individuals without reference to the broader political context (Bracken, 1998; Kleinman, 1995). This argument has become even more significant with the globalization of PTSD. Following what Didier Fassin defines as "humanitarian psychiatry" (2008: 534), researchers have examined how, in non-Western conflict areas lacking assistance infrastructures, humanitarianism has moved from responding to the "basic needs" of human survival to professional therapy aimed at psychological issues. Thus, PTSD serves as a magnifying glass for observing different forms of suffering around the globe (Breslau, 2004; Fassin and Rechtman, 2009).

For example, the introduction of the PTSD discourse into Haiti between 1995 and 2000, a period characterized by the regime's instability and an attempted military coup, created new relationships between the humanitarian aid organizations, their sources of funding, and local residents. Thus, the professionals authorized aid mainly based on biographical events that had caused trauma, and the very nature of a diagnosis allowed access to material assistance as well as national and international recognition (James, 2004).

In another setting, following the October 2002 terror attacks in Bali, Indonesia, the U.S. Agency for International Development introduced the clinical tool of PTSD through the work of mental health professionals who treated hundreds of the island's residents. Henceforth, PTSD became part of the local vocabulary used to describe the local suffering. However, this process was not free of social negotiation and political implications. The residents of Bali were ambivalent about professional intervention. Although PTSD became an important instrument for gaining treatment for their mental distress, some residents perceived it as a repressive discourse that overshadowed alternative narratives. They described their suffering as being rooted in Bali's unacknowledged political discourse, which differed from the apparently universal PTSD discourse (Dwyer and Santikarma, 2007).

As with PTSD, the extension of the primary trauma to significant others, usually termed "secondary trauma," has also been examined critically from an anthropological perspective. Arguing that the transmission of trauma "must be understood as more than just the contagiousness of psychological symptoms" (Dickson-Go'mez, 2002: 416), researchers have described the various sociocultural ways in which traumatized memories are passed on to subsequent generations and reinterpreted through different narrative strategies. For example, under the guidance of a therapist, descendants of Holocaust survivors use the clinical definition of PTSD as a crucial means of constructing a new self-identity as second-generation victims (Kidron, 2004). In Santiago, Chile, between the years 2000 and 2004, and in 2009, researchers examined how gender expectations shaped the aftermath of traumatic experiences in terms of the individual's perception of recovery. Based on the story of one of the Chilean women, the research exposes how a lifetime of gender-based violence and suffering was deeply embedded within the cultural, political, and social context in which she lived (Parson, 2010).

Trauma, PTSD, and other subcategories, such as secondary trauma, therefore, have become a "taken-for-granted dimension of humanitarian assistance on a global level" (Breslau, 2004: 114). The mental suffering of individuals has become the focus, while broader sociopolitical questions are pushed aside. Vanessa Pupavac (2001), for example, critically analysed this process by referring to it as "therapeutic governance." She claims that the mere description of a given community or population as having experienced conflict is sufficient for international agencies to deem them to be suffering from PTSD and in need of psychosocial assistance. Through the "pathologisation of distress" (Pupavac, 2001: 5), a new form of international assistance takes place based on social risk management. While focusing on individual feelings as their reference point, trauma experts may obscure the original sources of conflict while blurring the political issues associated with it.

However, in addition to the medicalization and depoliticization of suffering, increasing global awareness caused the diagnostic category of trauma to become entangled with local systems of meanings (Breslau, 2004; Fassin and Rechtman, 2009). Under this second theoretical direction, anthropologists have examined how, in non-Western countries, the disorder has overlapped with local experiences of distress. In trauma stories of Ethiopian refugees in Somalia, for example, issues of injustice and social rift, rather than private emotional suffering, are prominent (Zarowsky, 2004). Similarly, distress narratives told by a formerly exiled communist militant and her daughter who were of low socio-economic status in Chile reveal that trauma, history, and memory were woven together and processed partly to negotiate a political-ethical position. They did not understand trauma in individual terms, but rather as a "dissonance of relations" nourished by the tension between the socialist language of the past and the neoliberal language of the present (Han, 2004). In Liberia after the civil war (1990–2003), humanitarian agencies transformed a culture-bound disorder named "Open Mole" into a local term for trauma. Later, it became a gateway diagnosis of PTSD-related mental illness, and the international experts considered how to classify it objectively as an experience of psychiatric disorder (Abramowitz, 2010).

The term "national trauma" provides an interesting illustration to how trauma and PTSD have been intersected by local and historical circumstances. In contrast to seeing trauma as a universal experience, this term describes the deep connection between mental distress and sociopolitical questions of national belonging. From a medical perspective, national trauma is a series of individual PTSD cases that reach a critical mass within a specific national context, therefore causing them to carry a symbolic meaning. For instance, after the September 11 attacks, researchers reported that indirect exposure to the events through the media or relatives led to the development of PTSD on a large scale (Silver et al., 2002).

At the same time, national trauma has been defined more broadly from a cultural perspective. Rather than based on diagnosed or anticipated individual psychopathology, under this perspective mental vulnerability and suffering have been tied to personal and collective experiences of identity. According to this idea, "cultural trauma occurs when members of a collective feel they have been subjected to a horrendous event that leaves indelible marks upon their group consciousness, marking their memories forever and changing their future identity in fundamental and irrevocable ways" (Alexander, 2004: 1). In post–Apartheid South Africa, for example, a new political identity of "national victim" was constructed by bringing individual suffering "into a public space where it could be collectivized and shared by all and merged into a wider narrative of national redemption" (Wilson, 2000: 80). Similarly, after the September 11 attacks, Young (2007) coined the term "PTSD of the virtual kind": American citizens were encouraged to think of themselves as "participant-observers in a traumatic event" (42), and the concept of "resilience" against trauma received special attention from researchers, clinicians, patients, and the wider public.

This study, therefore, addresses two interrelated anthropological accounts that stem from the intense interplay between the global and local spheres surrounding the professional management of trauma. While the first one focuses on how trauma has become a tool within the humanitarian discourse for the sake of identifying the "pure victims in general" (Malkki, 1996: 378), the second analyses how the same clinical construct of trauma has turned out to be another means for reassuring cultural and national boundaries.

Israel is an ideal case study for such an ethnographic inquiry. Upon its establishment in 1948, Israel defined itself as a Jewish and democratic state, combining the qualities of a pioneer mentality together with collectivist tendencies. As a result, whereas Jewish immigrants become Israeli citizens upon arrival and receive substantial benefits, the Palestinians who have remained within Israel's recognized borders since the 1948 War have found themselves in an inequitable situation. While Israel has incorporated this population into the body politic of the state as citizens and provided them with basic rights, such as representation in governmental institutions, Palestinians have been excluded from the Jewish-Israeli national "we" and are frequently considered, explicitly and implicitly, a subversive group. Over the years, the Palestinians have suffered ongoing discrimination, from an inferior position in the local labour market and from the poor allocation of resources for health and education. Furthermore, in addition to this ethno-national stratification, another bitter political and social axis in power relations has developed in Israel between the right and left wings of the Jewish population, and between Jewish immigrants from Eastern Europe and Jewish immigrants from North Africa (Kimmerling, 1993; Shafir and Peled, 2002; Rabinowitz, 2001).

Thus, while the globalized concept of trauma became an integral part of the clinical expertise in Israel and focused on the individual, the local experts have often been confronted with the broader sociopolitical context, with all the dynamics of power evolved within it, when addressing post-traumatic symptoms. As a result, the Israeli mental health experts faced a new array of dilemmas, challenges, and tensions, which provide the point of departure for this book.

The Israeli Case: Trauma and Nation-building

Many years ago, at the time of the War of Liberation, in Kibbutz Ma'ale Hachamisha, beneath the famous cemetery of the Harel Brigade, at the height of the battle over Jerusalem, a rather unique group of combat soldiers, whose comrades called them the "Degs" (from "degenerate"), gathered together. These were soldiers whose spirits had waned. Their comrades and commanders, who would be facing death at night, perceived them as a bunch of cowards, deserters, shirkers, impostors trying to avoid the nocturnal battle.

– Yuval Neriya, *In the Shadow of War* (1994: 5)

The above description by clinical psychologist Yuval Neriya perfectly illustrates the attitude of both the IDF (Israeli Defense Forces) and large segments of Israeli society towards mental suffering caused by the 1948 War. The "perspective of the truth that can teach us about the real effects of the war in the mental field" (Neriya, 1994: 5) was not heard.

Given the reality of protracted military conflict, in which Israel has been involved since its inception, many Israelis routinely process military and "security" considerations as integral aspects of everyday life. The Zionist perception of the precariousness of Jewish existence as a defenceless minority in the diaspora, which was nightmarishly substantiated in the Holocaust, and the threats posed to Israel's existence during its formative years, gave birth to strong pressures for heroism among Israeli men (Lieblich, 1978). A unique system of cultural meaning, which Kimmerling (1993) called "cognitive militarism,"[2] evolved during the state's formative years, and canonized the myth of heroism. The consensus that the IDF was an indispensable safeguard of individual and national survival was a basic tenet of Israelis' cognitive militarism. This ideological background fostered a collective mood that downplayed the psychic toll of war and military violence and stigmatized their emotional manifestations. Thus, while Israel has strong ties to the global communities in the West, particularly to the U.S., in the fields of advanced scientific research and clinical expertise, facing core national values and the adversity of ongoing violent conflict have played an essential role in shaping the professional attitude towards mental vulnerability.

---

2 Kimmerling (1993) defines cognitive militarism as a latent state of mind, which arises "when the civilian leaders ... regard the primary military and strategic considerations as being self-evidently the only or the predominant considerations in most of the societal and political decisions or priority ordering" (206).

During the 1948 War, despite the imminent threat of destruction and the high number of casualties, psychological casualties were marginalized. An ideologically informed reluctance to acknowledge the possibility of a psychological breakdown among Israeli soldiers was the reason for this marginalization. This bias, reinforced by poor medical administration and scarce psychiatric resources, made it easy to ignore combat stress reactions altogether, or to view them as stemming from "cowardice" or "lack of motivation," as the quote above by Neriya (1994) demonstrates. Psychological casualties that could not be disregarded were treated in well-insulated psychiatric units, shrouded in secrecy, and irrevocably released from service upon recovery. Those who remained traumatized, therefore, found it hard to be officially recognized as disabled war veterans.

Psychological casualties became even more difficult to assess during the 1967 War. A nascent military mental health system was already in existence when the war broke out, but the recognition threshold of combat stress reactions remained high. From the Israeli perspective, an alarming waiting period preceded the dramatic trajectory of the 1967 War, followed by a blitzkrieg that ended with an overwhelming victory. These events created a climate of national euphoria that bolstered the myth of heroism. Under such circumstances, combat stress reactions were marginalized once again.

The myth of heroism, and with it the disregard and denial that had concealed combat stress reactions from the public eye in the preceding wars, extensively eroded during the 1973 War. Following the utter surprise and confusion at the onset of the war, the military defeats in the first days of fighting and the heavy toll of casualties were etched onto the national consciousness as a massive trauma. The ensuing sense of disillusionment and vulnerability instilled in the Israeli public a greater readiness to face the dire psychological consequences of combat duty. This readiness was only partially evident in the army. While the military mental health system was flooded with massive waves of psychological casualties, high-ranking officers still clung to the belief that paying medical attention to these problems might amplify rather than attenuate them.

During the First Lebanon War of 1982, a confluence of factors made psychological breakdown in battle more visible. Four factors have contributed to Israel's growing awareness of the psychological problems related to battles and their long-term effects: (1) the "de-glorification process" that stained Israel's wars since the 1970s, (2) the heated controversy over the necessity, scope, and outcome of each war, (3) the intense contact between the combat and non-combat population, and (4) the introduction of PTSD to the third edition of the DSM-III (Solomon, 1993).

The Palestinian uprising in the Occupied Territories, known as the First Intifada of 1987–9, further sensitized public opinion in Israel to security-based trauma. The factors contributing to this process included two elements: (1) the widening circles of Israeli civilians caught in the spiral of violence, and (2) the escalating controversy over the moral justification for military control of the Territories and the resulting violent clashes with Palestinian civilians. The psychological cost of the occupation became an oft-discussed subject in Israel's public arenas, from political institutions and the media to artistic creations and professional conferences (Gal, 1990).

However, the Second Intifada, which broke out in October 2000, marked another turning point in the discourse of PTSD in Israel. In contrast to the First Lebanon War of 1982 and the First Intifada of 1987–9, the Second Intifada was defined as "a war of no choice," but this time it was a new kind of war:

> A series of hundreds of terror attacks, to which the Israeli population has been exposed, created a unique type of [mental] stress ... People were injured and murdered while walking on the city sidewalks, driving in their cars, or even while sleeping in their beds ... The victims of the terror attacks were soldiers, civilians, grownups, the old, women and children, discotheque-goers and ultra-Orthodox [*haredim*], Israeli natives, new immigrants, Arabs and foreign workers. (Somer and Bleich, 2005: 10–11)

As this description by psychiatrists Eli Somer and Avi Bleich indicates, the common perception among mental health experts referred to the threat of terror by Palestinian organizations, such as Hamas and Islamic Jihad, as cutting across social categories, ostensibly blind to any differences between women and men, Jews and Arabs, soldiers and civilians, native Israelis and those who had just arrived.[3] This perception helped solidify a new trend in research regarding civilian trauma in the context

---

3 According to the Foreign Ministry data, in 2000 there were four suicide terror attacks in which 43 people were killed; in 2001, there were 35 terror attacks in which 204 people were killed; in 2002, the number of terror attacks reached its peak, 60, in which 451 people were killed; in 2003, there were 26 terror attacks in which 210 people were killed; in 2004, there were 15 terror attacks in which 117 people were killed; and in 2005, there were 7 terror attacks in which 55 people were killed.

of conflict, the harbingers of which had already appeared during the First Gulf War (e.g., Milgram, 1994). The expanded application of PTSD to Israeli citizens was the result of studies that were conducted on the mental effects of terror events on various groups in Israel (see in Somer and Bleich, 2005), and the mental effects of the September 11 attacks (Danieli, Brom, and Sills, 2005; Knafo, 2004). Based on previous findings regarding the terror events in the U.S. (Silver et al., 2002; Young, 2007), the local clinicians concluded that direct exposure to terror events was not necessary and that indirect exposure could suffice to cause the appearance of PTSD symptoms (Bleich, Gelkopf, and Solomon, 2003).[4] They claimed that the heightened risk of developing the disorder required therapists to be much more involved than in the past in treating the mental fallout from the traumatic event in large institutions, such as the educational system and hospitals. This new professional direction, they explained, could promote among caregivers and the public an increased awareness of the existence of PTSD and the need for those experiencing it to receive mental health aid (Somer and Bleich, 2005).

The professional management of trauma and PTSD in Israel, therefore, depicts a medical undertaking that has been shaped by a powerful national narrative repeatedly challenged in its clinical scope by social, political, and religious dynamics of power. This unique undertaking is occurring in a society where two contradictory sociopolitical belief systems exist side by side: individualism and collectivism. The tense relations that have developed over the years between the factions representing each of these sociopolitical belief systems have shaped the raison d'être of the State of Israel and marked the social boundaries of the national collective. This dichotomy, in turn, influences and is influenced by the professional attitude towards emotional vulnerability in the context of the Arab–Israel conflict.

Studies from a sociological and anthropological perspective that researchers have conducted in the last two decades have identified this

---

4 Research by Avraham Bleich, Mark Gelkopf, and Zehava Solomon, published in *JAMA* in 2003, presents the most noteworthy empirical data. Through a telephone survey among a representative national sample of 512 households, conducted in April–May 2002, they examined the psychological effects of the continuing terror on Israel's citizens. The findings showed that, although more than half of those surveyed had not been exposed personally to a terror event and did not know anyone close to them who had, 76.7 per cent reported at least one PTSD-related symptom.

new professional approach towards trauma. Through analysis of professional and journalistic texts, for example, Edna Lomsky-Feder and Eyal Ben-Ari point to how the definition of trauma has become strongly established in Israeli public discourse. Trauma, they argue, is an efficient contemporary tool for normalizing the experience of war into the routine life of Israel citizens, because the public defines trauma as apolitical and neutral (Lomsky-Feder and Ben-Ari, 2011). At the same time, researchers argue that the approach to trauma is for the most part ideological and politically committed (Plotkin-Amrami, 2013). The Israeli experts, it has been claimed, tend to emphasize the suffering of Jewish-Israeli citizens while paying little heed to the distress of the Palestinian-Israeli citizens and portraying the Palestinians of the Occupied Territories as perpetrators of terror (Brunner, 2006).

While the current research should be seen as a part of this critical analysis of the contemporary professional approach towards trauma, it differs in that is based on a rich, prolonged, and multi-sited ethnography at two local NGOs, NATAL and ITC. By providing specific descriptions of the professional work of both NGOs during the last decade, I examine how two interrelated dimensions have been evolved around the new professional sensitivity to mental vulnerability under the current security circumstances of Israel: first the political and then the pragmatic. In the *political dimension,* I explore the social relations that emerge among mental health experts (including psychiatrists, clinical psychologists, psychotherapists, and social workers), representatives of state agencies, donors, community leaders, marketing teams, and local residents from different ethnic and socio-economic backgrounds. All of these social players have become involved in an ongoing negotiation over the meaning of trauma, what is at stake when facing existential threats in the north or in the south of the country, and over the allocation of financial and organizational resources for the sake of providing aid. Following the political dimension is the *pragmatic dimension,* in which I explore the specific forms of communication and the types of interventions that have developed in various settings in Israel. I claim that the Jewish-Israeli experts have sketched out new, broader, and more flexible definitions of traumatic injury from the iconic definition of PTSD, blurring the distinction between the "pathological" and the "normal."

Through these two processes, the professional management of trauma and PTSD has changed dramatically. Not only have local experts extended their scope of activity from treating clinical symptoms borne by individuals to fortifying entire communities, but also a new way of speaking about mental vulnerability and national belonging has developed in contemporary Israel. This new way stems from a combination of individual psychopathology and collective markers of the Jewish-Israeli identity. While traditionally trauma and PTSD were clinical concepts familiar only to the mental health experts dealing with it and relevant only to the small minority diagnosed with it, throughout the chapters of the book it will become clear how those clinical definitions have been transformed into new categories of identity, raising new tensions and contradictions, new dynamics of power, as well as new forms of dialogue.

Structure of the Book

The book is divided into seven chapters. The first three chapters deal with the political dimension of trauma in Israel. They describe the establishment of new organizational platforms for treating traumatic injuries under the current security circumstances of Israel. This description revolves around the ongoing negotiation between the various social players within and outside those platforms, while analysing the relationships that developed between them. The last four chapters deal with the pragmatic dimension of trauma. These chapters describe the new definitions and subdefinitions of trauma the experts have expanded from the original classification of PTSD while extending their scope of intervention from the individual to the community, and to the entire nation.

The first chapter deals with the birth of two organizations that are dedicated to working on behalf of the diagnostic category of trauma, but only one is exclusively tied to Israel's military conflict with the Palestinians and the neighbouring Arab states. How do the local experts distinguish post-traumatic symptoms that have developed in the context of military service and terror attacks from those that have developed following car accidents or sexual abuse? Moreover, what happens when those experts, whose training focused on treating soldiers from the Israeli army and Jewish citizens exposed to Palestinian terror attacks, find themselves confronted by atypical victims of trauma? Ethnographic cases of such victims include a young woman from an illegal Jewish settlement in the Occupied Territories who developed PTSD when she resisted forced evacuation by the Israeli security forces, and Arabs living in northern Israel exposed to repeated rocket fire during the Second Lebanon War.

The second chapter is devoted to the unique relationships that have developed between the Jewish-Israeli trauma experts and the Jewish-American donors. This chapter examines the creative attempt to make traumatic injury accessible, even more attractive, for donors in order to elicit recognition, compassion, and money. This intersection became even more intense when it developed into a practical negotiation between therapists and donors regarding financial allocation for mental aid under the changing security circumstances of the Arab–Israeli conflict.

The third chapter presents the expansion of the social circle surrounding trauma and PTSD, from experts and donors to marketing advisers. I analyse a debate over NATAL's name and logo being represented in three languages (Hebrew, English, and Arabic) and examine a somewhat conflicted production of a documentary film while searching for the most effective ways to represent trauma and PTSD in the context of the conflict. By doing so, I explore how three Israelis became "talents of trauma": a young woman who worked as a security guard at a mall and was subjected to a terror attack; a man who worked as a firefighter and rescued the wounded from a terror attack; and a bereaved mother who lost her son in a military operation in the Gaza Strip.

The fourth chapter focuses on how civic trauma experts from NATAL have returned to the original context in which the professional awareness of traumatic injuries had started to develop: the IDF. I describe four professional practices those experts have applied for the sake of expanding the relevancy of trauma and PTSD to Israeli soldiers: (1) clinical therapy among veterans suffering from severe PTSD, (2) documentation of prisoners of war narratives, (3) quantitative and qualitative research of soldiers in the Second Intifada, and (4) outreach to veterans of the Second Lebanon War. In doing so, I show how the clinical disorder of PTSD has become a new means of framing the moral dilemmas that military service poses not only to the Israeli soldiers themselves but also to all of Israeli society.

The fifth chapter describes the first expansion of the professional treatment from primary trauma, PTSD, to a secondary trauma. Based on research involving participant observation at a support group for women married to men diagnosed as suffering from PTSD, I examine how the professional responses to the men's PTSD and the attempt to avoid the development of secondary trauma among the women intersect with gender issues of sex, intimacy, and power struggles in the kitchen, the living room, and the bedroom.

The sixth chapter presents a further expansion of PTSD as a clinical diagnostic category (concerned with the primary and secondary levels of the disorder) into a new arena: at-risk groups. I examine four professional interventions among community members who presumed to be especially vulnerable to developing post-traumatic symptoms: workshops for right-wing, ultra-Orthodox Jewish settlers; training sessions for Bedouin social workers; a seminar for bereaved Druze parents; and aid intervention for secular Jewish children on a kibbutz. Through this process, I uncover the dynamic between the clinical orientation of the trauma experts and the everyday life of the aid recipients.

The seventh chapter deals with the most dramatic expansion of trauma therapy in contemporary Israel: from diagnosis and treatment of individual symptoms to a disorder that can be anticipated and prevented by fortifying the entire community. By describing the "resilience program" that was implemented in the southern town of Sderot in response to the Qassam rocket attacks, I analyse how the experts began to manage the entire community based on three innovative professional practices: mobile clinics, haven rooms, and resilience workshops. In describing each one of them, I shed light on how the professional treatment of trauma has become intertwined with ethnic, economic, and political hierarchies.

The eighth and concluding chapter argues that the new professional approach to mental vulnerability under the current security circumstances of Israel has not necessarily been tied to "hard," evidence-based findings. Instead, a metamorphosis in how trauma and PTSD are addressed and treated has taken place, which has eventually led to a new therapeutic contract around mental vulnerability in Israel. Following the current anthropological accounts dealing with the globalization of trauma, I analyse how this new contract has become enmeshed within the local individualism and collectivism belief systems, leaving both aid providers and receivers to deal with trauma while treading cautiously around sensitive clinical and political issues.

Chapter One

Birth of Agencies, Birth of an Interpretative Framework

In the last two decades, two new organizational platforms have been established in Israel for the purpose of offering professional treatment to trauma victims in the context of the Arab–Israeli conflict: NATAL (the Israel Center for Victims of Terror and War), and the umbrella organization ITC (the Israel Trauma Coalition). Both of these organizations have tried to pave their own professional paths alongside two state agencies that have been operating in Israel since the mid-1960s: the Disabled Rehabilitation Division of the Ministry of Defense treats trauma victims of military service, and the National Insurance Institute assists victims of terror attacks. The senior trauma experts from NATAL and ITC attempted to carve out a professional niche for themselves during the Disengagement Plan of August 2005 and the Second Lebanon War of July 2006. These events serve as case studies to analyse how, under the new wings of NATAL and ITC, the boundaries of trauma kept changing, and how trauma and PTSD eventually turned into fluid concepts characterized by both flexibility and ambiguity.

NATAL: Sketching Out a Clinical Agenda

[At the beginning] nobody came to NATAL. NATAL was established in 1998 and it very much wanted to treat national trauma but, unfortunately, national trauma refused to be treated.

> – Dr. Danny Iger, clinical psychologist and
> one of NATAL's directors, 7 January 2005

The above description of NATAL's initial failure to establish itself as a necessary organization providing aid is a good place to begin pinpointing the politics that developed around trauma in the context of the conflict. The tension Dr. Danny Iger described between the assumption that Israel's citizens were suffering from trauma, the "national trauma" NATAL "very much wanted to treat," and the absence of patients, or as Iger put it, the refusal of the national trauma "to be treated," should be understood in light of what occurred in the months prior to launching the NGO. During this period, NATAL's founding team established a particular meaning of security-based trauma. That process was identified mainly with Dr. Yossi Hadar, a son of Holocaust survivors, who had served as a doctor in the 1973 War and later specialized in psychiatry. Co-founder of NATAL, Hadar held that the uniqueness of this agency lay in being a civilian NGO designed to bridge the gap that had opened up between Israel and its soldiers. In an interview, Hadar's spouse explains:

> Yossi represents trauma walking on two legs ... He felt that as a child, the State of Israel had been a counter-experience to the events of the Holocaust ... And that illusion was completely shattered for him during the 1973 War ... He was moments away from falling into Syrian captivity, and I think that was the first basis for his trauma at a national level; the Big Mama that is called the State of Israel was shattered for him ... His take on NATAL was that trauma on a national level concerns a very primary feeling of abandonment, like a baby abandoned by his mother – that the state didn't protect him. (Interview, 15 March 2005)

Hadar traced trauma to the rupture between the state, "the Big Mama," and those who had been drafted into service, the "babies" it had abandoned. However, the relative quiet in the Arab–Israeli arena in the year of NATAL's founding, 1998, made that vision difficult to achieve, as Iger aptly described. The absence of patients, together with the sudden death of Hadar from leukemia, led some of NATAL's founding team members to doubt the drawing power of the moral engine with which the NGO embarked. A variety of other types of trauma quickly arose as possible "candidates" for treatment. Tammi Sade, for example, a clinical psychologist and one of the founding team members, recalled: "I thought that maybe we should convert [the NGO's work] to treating accident victims, who are a neglected and abandoned public" (interview, 27 January 2005). Sade's idea, with which others concurred, of dealing with "PTSD stemming from killing that we are causing to ourselves" was rejected. The efforts to focus on a certain type of traumatic injury, PTSD due to the Arab–Israeli conflict, as an exclusive locus of professional treatment rather than a traumatic incident such as a car accident, made it necessary to provide further explanations that would justify this mode of action. Sade herself characterized this traumatic injury based on its "social aspect":

> There is a thing about the feeling of a mission – it's something that's beyond the individual. I think that in rape, women don't feel at that moment that they represent the feminine gender, and the thing with [national] trauma is that people represent something … It's madness with justification, madness with meaning. It's not just some poor fellow who genetically is in that percentage of the population that gets schizophrenia … There is a feeling of mission, a feeling of collective, a feeling of state, society, community, place, family, and of Judaism and roots. (Interview, 15 March 2005)

The above remarks by Sade, alongside similar statements by many other NATAL therapists, shed light on the "standard hallmark" they formed from the iconic clinical definition of PTSD and placed at the centre of the NGO's professional agenda: a traumatic injury related to action performed by an individual on behalf of a collective. Like Hadar before them, Sade and her colleagues identified that injury at the interface between the citizen and the nation: the individual was striving to secure the existence of the state, but while acting as an emissary of the state, the individual became a victim. Therefore, his suffering was distinct from that of the woman who had been raped, the man injured in a traffic accident, and the mentally ill, as they were not emissaries of the state. The state did not send them into the street, onto the road, or into the segment of the population that suffers from a certain disease. However, whereas Hadar referred to the victim's abandonment by the state as the locus of the traumatic injury, Sade and others emphasized the individual as having been wounded on *behalf* of the state, not *by* the state. The fact that the individual is part of "Judaism and roots" is what gives emotional charge and traumatic potential to a particular event.

Thus, the drafting of the basic definition around which the therapeutic work was to be organized prompted a delicate but highly meaningful turning point away from a subversive perception of trauma to a more conservative one. While Hadar's vision was an invitation to reveal a mental injury originating from high levels of anger and protest against the state, under the revised meaning of PTSD the individual's memory was bound up with the collective memory (Halbwachs, 1992), and vice versa; and the individual's mental injury was tied to the injury to the state, and vice versa. "Even though traffic accidents are a terrible thing that I think causes enormous damage, still there is no feeling that it harms the collective existence, that it harms the state, that the state will cease to exist," explained Sa'ar Uzieli, director of the NATAL clinical team. "During the difficult period of terror attacks [of the Second Intifada], people expressed that feeling: that we won't live here, that we'll be expelled, that we'll be beaten, and then the identification [with the traumatic circumstances] is much greater" (interview, 28 March 2005).

Professor Avi Bleich, a senior psychiatrist and the chair of the NATAL steering committee, further honed that concept. Bleich (a reserve colonel) served as head of the IDF mental health department, as former chair of the Israel Psychiatric Association, and is a current manager of one of Israel's largest psychiatric hospitals. Based on his many years of experience in various therapeutic settings, Bleich explained the exceptionality of PTSD in the context of the conflict:

> [It is] a trauma, a large part of whose unique aspects of its "impact" stems from your being not just a person who lives here [but also] you're an Israeli and a Jew ... All of these things carry within them, at least theoretically, unique characteristics of trauma, which are to some extent part of the Israeli-Jewish identity in the Land of Israel ... Does this traumatization have, for example, different phenomenological aspects from a trauma victim in a Bronx ghetto or from an English veteran of the Falklands? That interests me much less. (Interview, 8 August 2005)

Uzieli's and Bleich's use of the Israeli Zionist narrative indicates how the fundamental distinction they made regarding security-based trauma injury in Israel, in contrast to other places, turned into a "clinical ideology" (Young, 1995: 199). The therapists developed a conceptual framework reliant on scientific, universal, and global knowledge related to the clinical disorder of PTSD. However, this conceptual framework also contained distinctive social and cultural components: in order to deal with the trauma, it considered the broader context of place, of national and religious belonging. It distinguished the victim's injury from that of a PTSD victim "in a Bronx ghetto" or of "an English veteran of the Falklands."

The NGO's formal statement reflects the two-pronged clinical agenda regarding security-based trauma located specifically in Israel:

NATAL was established on the assumption that national trauma victims are unique and should be distinguished from victims of other traumatic experiences such as car accidents, family violence, or rape. The uniqueness stems from the combination of the posttraumatic stress syndrome of these casualties and the social, public, and national context in which the harmful event occurred. These individuals have paid, and keep paying, the toll for the road we are all taking, and we believe that Israeli society is being tested for its ability to extend a helping hand to them. NATAL was established to be part of this helping hand. (NATAL, www.natal.org.il)

NATAL's agenda is, therefore, a creative attempt to interweave the apparently incompatible discourses of the "therapeutic" and the "national." The opening declaration insisting on a therapeutic ethos devoid of political considerations coincides with the globalized notion of PTSD as a biomedical concept that underlies the psychological effects of suffering (Breslau, 2004; Kleinman, 1995; Young, 1995). Since, by definition, the trauma is situated in a "social, public, and national context," the apolitical orientation appears untenable. A distinctive moral sentiment is inherently attached to security-based trauma, which relates to an implicit violation of the agreement between the state and its citizens. Whether a soldier collapses in battle or a civilian is injured in a suicide bombing, the context of their suffering makes them representatives of the Israeli collective and holds the state morally accountable for them.

Under this professional agenda, therefore, NATAL's therapists have had to manoeuvre between clinical concerns and the sociopolitical dynamics of everyday life from the very start. They provided therapeutic treatment of the "self," but with the understanding that the victim's pathological memories were interconnected with the collective and its national ethos. The therapists situated themselves, without necessarily meaning to, on the seam between the global and the local domains and between the private and the public spheres. Consequently, these therapists had to walk the line between sensitive clinical and sociopolitical issues.

The Disengagement Plan: Controversy over the Basic Equation

The ongoing effort to define the boundaries of NATAL's clinical agenda was revealed when the NGO's therapists dealt with an unusual event in the context of the Arab–Israeli conflict: the Disengagement Plan of August 2005. Following the Israeli government's decision in October

2004, the plan forced the evacuation of 8,600 National Orthodox Jewish settlers from their homes in the Gaza Strip and the West Bank, most of whom identified with the right wing. While the vast majority of the Israeli public strongly supported the plan, the settlers protested violently against it under the slogan "One Jew doesn't evict another."

This profound disagreement represents the tense relations between the right and left wings in Israel. A deep social boundary divides these groups, especially regarding the religious nature of Israel as a Jewish-democratic state. This boundary is also evident in relation to the actual ability to reach some kind of political agreement with the Palestinians and the neighbouring Arab states. The focus is primarily on the Jewish settlements established in the Gaza Strip and the West Bank after the 1967 War. The new National Orthodox leadership claims their settlement project in the Occupied Territories is a continuation of the Zionist movement's pre-statehood settlement drive, as well as a contemporary fulfilment of the divine command to "redeem the land." Even though the Israeli government has always promoted the establishment of the settlements, they have become the embodiment of ardent right-wing Zionists. Small enclaves were established under heavy military protection, especially within the impoverished Palestinian region of Gaza, sparking a constant, bitter political debate (Kimmerling, 1993; Shafir and Peled, 2002).

In the political atmosphere after the Israeli government publicly disclosed the Disengagement Plan, several local trauma experts tried to warn of the development of PTSD symptoms among the Jewish settlers that would result from the expected forced evacuation. However, one local NGO, MaHUT, took this activity to a new level. MaHUT is an aid centre that was established during the 1980s in the West Bank by National Orthodox mental health therapists, most of whom lived in the Occupied Territories. The NGO's aid discourse has merged the political narrative of the Israeli right wing with the professional discourse of PTSD, claiming that living in the Jewish settlements created "ongoing stress," which "requires expertise, awareness, initiative and professional activity."[1]

This professional rationale was clearly apparent from the beginning of the public debate in Israel regarding the Disengagement Plan. Based

---

1 See MaHUT's website, http://www.shomron.org.il/?CategoryID=571, last accessed 14 May 2013.

on their expertise, but no less on their strong political identification with the Jewish settlers – being settlers themselves – MaHUT's practitioners estimated that 15 per cent to 30 per cent of the evacuees would suffer from PTSD symptoms. Therefore, they sought to raise awareness among their colleagues – most of them middle-class, secular Jews associated with the left wing (see Berman, 2003) – about the importance of public empathy and professional aid intervention for the settlers. For example, three months before the evacuation, Miriam Fogel, the head of MaHUT, was invited to speak about the mental state of the settlers at a meeting of young practitioners from the NATAL hotline. She explained:

> The [disengagement] plan refers to thirty-three small settlements, isolated and threatened by terrorism. There is the trauma of deportation, and [of] meeting the society to which you belong, and the feeling that no one understands and nobody wants to hear … It's like soldiers returning from captivity or Holocaust survivors … This plan is a historic decision, a very cruel act. (5 May 2005, Field Notes)

Clearly, Fogel tried to depoliticize the settlers' distress. Her explanation gave no reference to the bitter controversy surrounding the political act of Jewish settlements in the Occupied Territories. Instead, she depicted the settlers as passive victims of trauma, like prisoners of war and Holocaust survivors, and identifies their mental vulnerability as being a result of two external threats: the ongoing Palestinian terror and the present Israeli government plan ("a very cruel act").

However, in line with the tense political debate, the hotline's practitioners did not fully accept Fogel's remarks. They responded to her explanation of the situation, as did those in charge:

HOTLINE PRACTITIONER 1: When I, as a mother, send my son as a soldier to evacuate this population, it's hard for me to feel a sense of common destiny [with them].

HOTLINE PRACTITIONER 2: We are talking here about a population that has been evacuated for ideological reasons. Do we as therapists have something to suggest to them? Are they going to make a switch from belligerence and anger to other emotions?

SA'AR UZIELI (CLINICAL PSYCHOLOGIST AND THE HEAD OF NATAL CLINICAL STAFF): We can speak about loss, about identity, pain, and grief … This is proper therapeutic work.

DR. ITAMAR BARNEA (NATAL'S CHIEF PSYCHOLOGIST): There is the
    question as to whether this issue belongs to the NATAL agenda, because
    it is between Jews. NATAL has defined itself around the Arab–Israeli
    conflict, and the question is a legitimate one ... but there is no doubt that
    [the evacuation] is a traumatic experience; this is a meaningful mental
    trauma. (5 May 2005, Field Notes)

As can be seen, NATAL senior experts agreed with Fogel's perception.
Contrary to the younger practitioners, who did not see the evacuation
as another manifestation of the ongoing trauma resulting from the
Arab–Israeli conflict, the senior experts focused on the evacuees' "loss,
pain, and grief." In doing that, they clearly extended their own scope of
professional activity, which was based on the equation of "we the Jews"
(the victim) versus "them the Arabs" (the perpetrators).

The dispute over the legitimacy of expanding the therapeutic work
in order to include the Disengagement Plan became even more intense
in the face of another evacuation of Jewish settlers. This one occurred
on a much smaller scale, but was no less politically controversial. In
February 2006, after a long legal battle, 10,000 Israeli soldiers and police
officers evacuated an illegal Jewish settlement named Amona, which
had been established in the Occupied Territories in 1997. During the
evacuation, the soldiers and police faced violent resistance by approxi-
mately 4,000 protesters, all of them National Orthodox Jews identified
with the right wing. The protesters sat in front of the homes, linking
arms and legs, and threw cinderblocks, metal pipes, rocks, and paint
bottles at the security forces, which responded by beating them with
truncheons and setting upon them with mounted troops. By the end of
the evacuation, 200 people had been injured, a quarter of them police
officers and the rest Jewish settlers. A few weeks later, the psychological consequences of this event landed on the agenda of NATAL. During
the monthly steering committee meeting, Sa'ar Uzieli, the head of the
clinical staff, shared with his colleagues what he perceived to be a professional dilemma:

SA'AR UZIELI: A few days ago I received a request to treat a young
    woman from Amona who developed post-traumatic stress disorder
    following their violent struggle against the evacuation. This is the first
    time it's [been] very difficult for me to decide ... If my son was there as a
    soldier and beat them, and maybe got beaten up, and now she comes as a
    "case" ... I guess she is really in distress.

DR. BERGER (CLINICAL PSYCHOLOGIST): If we do not express our opinion on the behaviour of one victim of trauma or another, it does not matter if this girl cracked the police officer's head. Her suffering is suffering and there is no question ... it is our duty to help.

SA'AR UZIELI: It's easier for me to treat an Arab gone wild on "Land Day" [*Yom H'adama* in Hebrew], than to treat someone gone wild in Amona.

PROFESSOR LEVIN (RESEARCHER): So, if there is a group of radical right-wing activists who want to blow up the Temple Mount [*Har HaBayit* in Hebrew], and on their way, one of them loses his hand and develops PTSD symptoms?

DR. BERGER: My answer – accept him.

SA'AR UZIELI: The question is, how will the Israeli public receive it, if one day we treat an Arab-Israeli suicide bomber's family because they are suffering from trauma? (26 April 2006, Field Notes)

After receiving a request to treat a young woman from an illegal Jewish settlement, NATAL senior experts considered different (potential) victims of trauma in the context of the Arab–Israeli conflict. Clearly, they were trying to base their professional attitude towards all of the victims on the "meritocracy of suffering" (Bob, 2002: 36), defining "those in need" on the basis of clinical criteria. However, when considering a young violent demonstrator from an illegal Jewish settlement, this challenged the perspective of the senior experts, revealing the sociopolitical context in which they sought to apply the diagnostic category of PTSD. Each of the events to which NATAL experts referred, from those that occurred in the past to those that might occur in the future, served as a symbolic marker of the ethno-national hierarchies that have developed within Israel. In addition to the bitter political disagreement between right and left wing, represented through the hypothetical event of blowing up the Temple Mount, there were two other events mentioned during the discussion: "Land Day," an annual protest against Israel's anti-Palestinian policies, and the situation of an Arab-Israeli suicide bomber. Both political events were presented as indicators of the tense relations between Jewish and Palestinian citizens of Israel (see Rabinowitz, 2001; Shafir and Peled, 2002).

Thus, although NATAL experts naturally used trauma and PTSD to articulate an array of distressing security-related experiences, they also cited the atmosphere of political relations in which the traumatic injury occurred as being relevant to the professional question of whether or not to provide mental aid. In many ways, their discussion represented a new method for implementing PTSD. Instead of the familiar process of excluding the political in favour of the medical and isolating the clinical from the social (see Bracken, 1998; Kleinman, 1995; Young, 1995), NATAL experts cross-referenced them as a new moral and pragmatic platform for their professional work.

ITC: Sketching Out an Aid Policy

In October 2001, a new NGO was established in Israel: ITC. An intensive year of terror attacks by militant Palestinian organizations led the founders of ITC to adopt NATAL's clinical agenda: an umbrella agency that aims to provide coordinated, long-term mental assistance to Israeli citizens in the context of the Arab–Israeli conflict. However, contrary to NATAL, the main force behind ITC was not a local one, but rather a social player outside of the state: the UJA-Federation. The Jewish philanthropists' well-known affinity for Israel (Silber, 2008) was evident with the outbreak of the Palestinian uprising in October 2000. Two months after the collapse of the peace talks between Israel and the Palestinian Authority at Camp David, Palestinian violence erupted both inside and outside Israel's recognized borders. Five days later, the UJA-Federation gave a few Israeli NGOs financial grants of tens of thousands of dollars to provide immediate aid intervention to Jewish citizens who had been exposed to Palestinian violence. Alongside NATAL, several notable NGOs also received donations, such as AMCHA (its name is the code word that helped survivors identify fellow Jews during the Holocaust), founded in 1987 to provide mental aid for Holocaust survivors and the second generation, for example, and ICMC (Israel Crisis Management Center, or SELAH in Hebrew), founded in 1993 to provide mental and practical aid to immigrants coping with unexpected tragedy.

However, as the violent events continued, the Jewish-American donors gained the impression that the lack of coordination between the local NGOs was reducing the effectiveness of aid intervention. As Hanna Brosh, one of the UJA-Federation's representatives, explained in her interview:

[Towards an additional series of financial grants] we wrote a clause that whoever receives a grant from us has to commit to participating in the Israel Trauma Coalition (ITC) ... That name was ours and the initiative was ours. What took shape later – that was ours too … because the money was ours. (Interview, 12 March 2006)

The change in the donors' position, from supporting local NGOs to establishing the new platform for mental aid that Brosh refers to, triggered an intensive modification in the NGOs' modes of activity. Contrary to their former tendency to engage with vulnerable groups that carry special significance in the Zionist narrative, and, as a result, in Israeli society (e.g., Holocaust survivors, immigrants, and veterans), and consistent with the process of globalization of PTSD (Breslau, 2004; Fassin and Rechtman, 2009), the donors drew fine distinctions within the entire Israeli population. The distinctions included seven consensual target groups in the professional therapy of PTSD: children, elderly, first responders, hospital workers, hotline volunteers, psychosocial teams, and practitioners working in primary medical care. However, contrary to other humanitarian agencies that operate on behalf of international human rights, here the donors shared religious identity and core national values with the local experts and aid recipients. As a part of these close relations, they took the liberty of reconnecting the aid discourse associated with trauma and PTSD with basic components of the Zionist narrative. Alongside the seven target groups based on accepted professional criteria, the donors and the experts mutually decided to establish two additional groups: immigrants and soldiers. Jewish immigration to Israel and military service represent two fundamental aspects of the Zionist ethos (Kimmerling, 1993; Shafir and Peled, 2002).

A one-page ITC document (September 2003) published a year after the official establishment of this new agency, and distributed among the ITC's members, governmental agencies, and municipal authorities, clarifies this unique agenda by elaborating on ITC's professional goals:

> Developing systematic and comprehensive prevention and treatment of trauma; promotion programs to assist the rehabilitation of trauma victims at the individual, family and community levels; gathering information and mapping needs of the Israeli population exposed to trauma and stress; providing information and educating the Israeli public regarding how to deal with trauma; promotion and implementation of national projects.

By focusing on professional efforts to identify and treat specific individuals who have developed symptoms of trauma, the experts and donors sought to base their aid authority on the strong legitimacy assigned to trauma as a scientific clinical category (Breslau, 2004; Fassin and Rechtman, 2009). However, in defining traumatic injury as an integral part of everyday life in Israel, the experts extended their scope of treatment from the individuals who were diagnosed with post-traumatic symptoms to "treating" the entire nation. Through goals such as "promotion and implementation of national projects" and "mapping the needs of the Israeli population," Israeli society as a whole became an object of intervention as well. Thus, like NATAL, ITC internalized the sociopolitical context of the traumatic injury into its aid discourse, which experts typically sought to push aside (see Bracken, 1998; Kleinman, 1995; Young, 1995). Although they operate independently of Israel's policy and the government's budget, defining themselves as dealing with trauma as a result of the political environment, ITC's experts and donors articulated their agenda in the scope of the nation-state. From the beginning, therefore, the basic equation of the Zionist narrative, "us Jews – them Arabs" (Bilu and Witztum, 2000; Kimmerling, 1993; Shafir and Peled, 2002), served as a moral guideline for their professional work.

However, as the shifting circumstances of the Arab–Israeli conflict challenged the clinical agenda formulated at NATAL, they also challenged the organizational mechanism established within ITC. It was again the Disengagement Plan that exposed the deep tension between the clinical concerns underlying trauma and the social circumstances of daily life in Israel. After the Disengagement Plan, the Second Lebanon War became the focus of debate.

The Evacuee Target Group: The Struggle for Empirical Validation

In October 2005, a few weeks after Israel implemented the Disengagement Plan, the question of mental assistance to those who had now become Jewish evacuees was raised during one of ITC's council meetings. ITC was considering whether to establish a distinct target group in order to deal with the evacuees' traumatic experience of their forced relocation. As opposed to the two new consensual target groups, soldiers and immigrants, any similar organizational acknowledgment regarding the Jewish settlers was the focus of constant dispute. A few months before the evacuation, ITC had made initial professional efforts to assess the mental condition of the settlers. As its CEO, Nurit Levin, explained:

We pay salaries for eight practitioners in order to reach out to settlers at-risk [of developing PTSD]. We concentrate especially on bereaved families: forty-eight families now have graves there, and our goal now is to map out their needs. (Interview, 8 June 2005)

By identifying the most vulnerable group among the settlers, the bereaved families who needed to transfer their relatives' graves to the centre of the country, Levin was hoping to elicit a legitimate, evidence-based decision to establish the target group. The procedures implemented by practitioners, such as "reaching out" or "mapping needs," were perceived as objective tools for managing this process (see Redfield, 2006). However, ITC's attempt to extend this process to the entire settler population failed. At an ITC council meeting three weeks after the evacuation, the CEO clarified:

In Israel, the political pressures ... We found ourselves in a situation that is not usual for professionals as the intermediaries between the settlers and the government. [In the last few weeks] we have introduced to the settlers and to the government ministries a therapeutic-community model for aid intervention ... Miriam [Fogel, the head of MaHUT] was supposed to gather the data [regarding each settlement and community] and present it. At the last moment, the settlers cancelled all the meetings and the process got stuck. (11 September 2005, Field Notes)

However, the efforts to gather information continued. At a council meeting held several weeks later, the CEO reported:

NURIT LEVIN (ITC CEO): The information isn't being given to us. They're unwilling to cooperate. There's a different language. They want money, job openings, and their own people!

REUVEN SEGEV (ITC SENIOR PSYCHOLOGIST): We shouldn't be involved at all in providing them mental aid! ... We're blowing the bugle, but there's nothing behind it! Eighty per cent [of them] don't need any [mental] assistance! ... The monopoly of the [evacuees'] representatives over the needs has to be broken!

HANNAH BROSH (DONORS' REPRESENTATIVE): Here's a kind of short-circuit, so we [should] perform a pilot [to screen needs] by ourselves, and [then] we'll tell [the philanthropists] what we've learned, because we don't want to be stuck in this checkmate. (16 October 2005, Field Notes)

The tension between the clinical narrative involving the diagnosis of PTSD and the Jewish settlers' political narrative is clear (see Abramowitz, 2010; Han, 2004; Zarowsky, 2004). Against ITC's attempt to medicalize their suffering, the Jewish settlers insisted on associating their hardship, not with the apolitical meaning of mental disorder, but rather with the ethno-national power struggles within Israel that were clearly exhibited during the implementation of the Disengagement Plan. Within the familiar, well-known classifications of Israel society, the middle-class, Eastern-European trauma experts were associated with the left wing in Israel. Therefore, the settlers demanded professional treatment from their "own people," accompanied by resources such as money and jobs.

Despite the settlers' refusal to cooperate with ITC and, as a result, the failure described above to "carry the full legitimacy of scientific knowledge" (Breslau, 2004: 114), a few weeks later a decision was made. While the media fostered a public atmosphere emphasizing the difficulties of the settlers in their new temporary homes, ITC's CEO announced the establishment of a new target group: evacuees. Fogel, the head of MaHUT, welcomed the decision: "We want to bring more people [to engage with this issue], and to increase power and knowledge" (interview, 25 April 2006).

ITC initiated various psychosocial aid interventions following the decision to establish the evacuee target group. However, the question regarding the validation of the settlers' suffering remained unresolved. At a council meeting held in May 2006, Fogel, as head of the new target group, presented a surprising request to her ITC colleagues:

MIRIAM FOGEL: We should draw up a document and address it [to government ministries], in order to give warning of the injustice and stupidity done to the evacuees!

DR. SHOSHANI (SENIOR PSYCHIATRIST): When you talk about injustice, what is that? Does it reflect distress? Needs? Who decides? Interested people? Something must be planned that can be brought as an objective finding that reflects needs!

DR. RUTH LIN (CLINICAL PSYCHOLOGIST): Hard data has to be presented, and not impressionistic, so it can be submitted as a professional paper.

DR. SHOSHANI (to Fogel): What suffering do you want to prove? (14 May 2006, Field Notes)

Fogel did not answer Shoshani, and her request was removed from the ITC agenda.

Nevertheless, Fogel's request was an additional effort to use the scientific, globalizing meaning of PTSD to reconnect to the public sphere, rather than create distance from it as experts usually do (Bracken, 1998; Kleinman, 1995; Young, 1995). ITC's apolitical position should have served, from her point of view, as a means of political advocacy. Nonetheless, the requests to present "hard data" (Dr. Lin) or to provide an "objective finding" that reflects "needs" (Dr. Shoshani) were an attempt to problematize the evacuees' position due to the absence of medical, evidence-based proof of their suffering.

The Arab Target Group: The Struggle for Professional Representation

The issue of the mental suffering of the Arab population in Israel cropped up on the ITC agenda for the very first time during the Second Lebanon War. Following the abduction of two Israeli soldiers in July 2006, Israeli air force and ground forces launched a massive attack along the Lebanese border, sparking a retaliatory barrage of missiles in northern Israel. Four weeks of missile attacks endangered the lives of those living in this area. Due to the absence of protective infrastructure and alarm systems, of the forty-four Israeli citizens killed during the war, almost half were Palestinian.

The exposure of Palestinian-Israelis to missile attacks raised a poignant question: Who at ITC should represent their distress and spearhead an intervention plan, if at all? During the Disengagement Plan, there was an organizational affiliation between the Jewish settlers and one of the NGOs connected to ITC – MaHUT. However, in the case of the Palestinian-Israelis, none of the NGOs had a similar connection with the victims. This was not an accident. Treating victims of Palestinian terrorists during the Second Intifada in 2000 had intentionally excluded this population from ITC's professional agenda. As a result, any negotiations regarding this population became very challenging.

At a council meeting a few days after the Second Lebanon War ended, without any prior discussion, ITC's CEO announced the foundation of a new target group: minorities. Some considered any discussion unnecessary due to the harsh outcome of the war. Immediately after the announcement, Vered Gal, a clinical psychologist and the representative of Community Stress Prevention Center (a Jewish NGO operating in northern Israel among the Jewish population exposed to missile attacks since the First Lebanon War), took responsibility for the new target group. After a short break in the meeting and a few phone calls, she made it clear that she intended to appoint Dr. Hassan Abu-Bakr, a clinical psychologist and Palestinian expert, to manage the target group. Abu-Bakr was a familiar figure in the Israeli mental health field. He had been born in northern Israel in the late 1950s and, based on his parents' experience of the 1948 War, took a political stance against Israel's discriminatory policy towards the Palestinians. Gal informed the council that in the wake of the war's events, Abu-Bakr was working to establish a new NGO, *Saned* (meaning "aid" or "support" in Arabic), to deal with "mental trauma in the Arab community." She went on to explain:

> VERED GAL: After all, the goal is for the desk to be managed by minorities and not by non-minorities.
>
> PROFESSOR COHEN (SENIOR PSYCHIATRIST): Is he [Abu-Bakr] accepted by the Arab population?
>
> VERED GAL: What do you mean? And are we all accepted by the Jewish population?! She is a Muslim; her assistant is Christian, the secretary Circassian. To this group we have added a Druze ... She is not on behalf of someone. She is apolitical.
>
> PROFESSOR COHEN (sarcastically): We are very apolitical, all of us.
>
> (27 September 2006, Field Notes)

In her response to Cohen's assumption that there could be a singular authentic representative of the Palestinians as a "native" population, Gal tried to grasp the stick at both ends. She tried to portray Abu-Bakr as "apolitical," and at the same time justify his position as a legitimate representative of the Palestinians' suffering by describing his ethno-national identity and his prospective cooperation with a variety of practitioners, each representing a different ethnic group that was also living in northern Israel (Druze, Christian, and Circassian). Cohen's cynical response ("We are very apolitical, all of us") exposed this paradox: using political terms in order to convince them of Abu-Bakr's apolitical stance.

At a council meeting held several weeks later, the professional transition from the clinical to the political became even more dramatic. Gal submitted to the council Abu-Bakr's request to change the name of the target group from "Minorities" to "Arabs." This was far from a merely technical issue. While the former referenced the numerical inferiority of the group (minorities versus majority) as an "objective" indicator of the power struggles between the two groups, the latter highlighted ethno-national difference (Arabs versus Jews). The request was greeted with silence. Gal then reiterated her original proposal to appoint Abu-Bakr to manage the new target group, adding, "As soon as he finishes establishing his NGO, it should become a full member of ITC." She continued her suggestion in the following exchange, introducing the new idea of an "attaché":

> VERED GAL: Maybe an NGO in the process of being established could be considered the sub-NGO of a senior NGO.
>
> DR. SHAVIT (PSYCHIATRIST): There is something improper about us deciding on the Arab sector!
>
> VERED GAL: I suggest there will be a "host NGO," and from our NGO there will be a representative to handle the issues of the Arab sector.
>
> ARIEL ARAD (ITC ADMINISTRATOR): I'm of the opinion that at this stage, I'm not sure that his group members will view his participation as a positive thing. It will look as if he is the minority, and there's a big majority here.
>
> VERED GAL: Let's find a mechanism that will make it possible to turn someone into an "attaché."
>
> DR. SHAVIT: He doesn't have to be an attaché – that's exactly their position in Israeli society!
>
> DR. HAIM KATZ (CLINICAL PSYCHOLOGIST): One of the NGOs can attach him, and he needs to trust the head of the target group to represent him. (27 September 2006, Field Notes)

As can be seen, the decision-making process with regard to adding Abu-Bakr as a member of the ITC came to an impasse. While the council reached agreement on the organizational representation of the Palestinians' distress under a new target group entitled "Arabs," the dilemma remained regarding its professional leadership. Although no one doubted Abu-Bakr's clinical skills, they perceived his ethno-national identity as a legitimate focus for professional negotiation. In line with the colonialist mindset hinted at from the beginning of the decision-making process, the majority of ITC members were of the opinion that Abu-Bakr and his NGO should be admitted to the council only in the position of "guest," "sub-NGO," or "attaché" of a senior Jewish NGO. Only one member argued that Abu-Bakr should be a full and legitimate member of ITC, but his argument was sociopolitically motivated: the inclusion of Abu-Bakr would serve as a professional "correction" to the political asymmetry.

Five months later, after a long professional "silence," Gal, the temporary head of the Arab target group, provided ITC council members with an unexpected update:

> [After the war] we submitted to ITC a request to receive funding to do research [among the residents in the north]. We have not received confirmation ... and we began the study alone ... The results are very clear. The difference is between Jews and Arabs. Seventy per cent of the Jewish population [were] evacuated from their homes to family relatives, but only 30 per cent of the Arabs could [be] evacuate[d] ... Consequently, the exposure to rockets and carnage was higher among the Arab population, and more than 80 per cent of those living in the affected area developed PTSD symptoms. (24 December 2006, Field Notes)

The findings presented by Gal revealed, once again, the vulnerable Palestinian position, in terms of both ethno-national power struggles (the absence of relatives who could host them during the war) and mental health (80 per cent developed PTSD symptoms). Ruth Lahav, a clinical psychologist, responded to ITC's initial refusal to fund the research:

> RUTH LAHAV: The ambiguity and confusion is very worrying ... I think [the research] is very important!
> DR. LEVIN (CLINICAL PSYCHOLOGIST): The results should not be for scientific publications, but a basis for planning aid policy ... Five months after the war and we still have not planned even one aid program! (24 December 2006, Field Notes)

After the presentation of the new data and the participants' reflexive criticism of their professional impotency with regard to the Palestinians' mental health, Gal went on to inform the council that Abu-Bakr was urgently promoting two aid intervention programs under the new Arab target group. The first was to provide professional training for Arab family physicians in the north in order to provide primary care to patients who might be suffering from mental trauma. The second was to offer similar training for teachers in Arab elementary schools. Surprisingly, ITC rejected the request. ITC's CEO claimed that Abu-Bakr should submit the proposed interventions for approval as part of the activities of two other target groups already established within ITC:

hospital workers and children. Shortly afterwards, it became clear that Abu-Bakr would not be joining ITC. In the ITC meetings that took place during those months, the CEO repeatedly explained that according to the organization's legal guidelines, joining the council was dependent on at least two years' experience and on "economic resilience." As a professional initiative in its infancy, *Saned* clearly did not meet the two criteria. Without financial resources and organizational backup, it was almost impossible for Abu-Bakr to succeed in his efforts, and the attempts to establish a new aid organization dedicated to the mental suffering of the Palestinians failed.

ITC's aid discourse, therefore, was left dangling between practical and ethical dilemmas. This coincided with the process of simultaneously using medical terms and then pushing them aside – namely, medicalization and demedicalization. Both NATAL and ITC established their authority on medical grounds, and senior psychiatrists held key positions in both of them, making this scientific aspiration actual. Yet, as non-governmental agencies operating in Israeli civil society, they had relative freedom to interpret the meaning of mental trauma as a consequence of political conflict. Unencumbered by strict government guidelines for receiving financial assistance from the state, both aid agencies have operated in a fairly flexible and fluid professional environment.

Conclusion

To conclude, the work of NATAL and ITC represented a new, non-traditional, and less conservative professional approach to the mental vulnerability of Israeli residents as they confronted the existential threat of the Arab–Israeli conflict. Against the historical tendency of Israeli authorities to minimize the significance of mental causalities as a result of the conflict (Bilu and Witztum, 2000; Solomon, 1993), both NATAL and ITC were expanding public perception of security-based trauma among both Israeli civilians and soldiers. Furthermore, as state agencies, the Ministry of Defense and the National Insurance Institute applied the definition of trauma based on a rigid set of clinical criteria. These agencies implemented diagnostic processes in keeping with specific legal and medical procedures. Against this background, NATAL and ITC, as non-governmental aid agencies, implemented a less stringent approach. This approach was based on a wider and more flexible use of the term trauma, while deliberately blurring the line between evidence-based diagnosis and general professional impressions. The agencies interpreted the term so as to be free from rigid clinical criteria or specific legal or medical procedures. By doing that, mental experts from both NATAL and ITC became engaged in critical change in the professional therapy of trauma in Israel: from treating a small percentage of individuals clinically diagnosed with traumatic symptoms to reinterpreting the entire narrative of Israel through the mental condition of trauma.

While both agencies incorporated trauma and PTSD into the Israeli context for identification of those in need, they also added sociopolitical markers to these clinical constructs. Thus, in addition to the target groups established based on universal criteria, such as "children" and "elderly," the donors and experts also decided to establish groups that represented dominant factions in the Zionist narrative, such as "soldiers" and "immigrants" (Kimmerling, 1993; Shafir and Peled, 2002). Later on, with controversy but with no less relevance, they added groups such as "evacuees" and "Arabs."

However, with regard to the two latter clinical-political target groups, ITC responded differently to the creation of each one. Despite the absence of statistical proof of their mental suffering, the Jewish settlers received substantial representation within ITC, through the leadership of MaHUT, alongside financial resources and aid intervention. In contrast, despite the preliminary data regarding the large number of individuals suffering from PTSD symptoms among the Palestinians, the ITC council excluded Abu-Bakr and the efforts to establish a Palestinian aid organization to lead the Arab target group failed. Furthermore, national logic influenced even the basic question as to whether or not the violent situations themselves, namely, the evacuation and the missile attacks during the Second Lebanon War, were legitimate reasons for ITC interventions. In order to sidestep the political controversy between the right and left wings, the suffering of the Jewish settlers was compared to that of Holocaust survivors and prisoners of war, two experiences which carry profound meaning in Israel (Bilu and Witztum, 2000; Kidron, 2004). On the other hand, it was only when 300,000 Palestinians fell victim to the same villain as the Jewish citizens, namely, Hezbollah, that they were deemed eligible to be moved from their controversial political position to a new, consensual position as "those in need." From this position, they received, for the very first time, organizational acknowledgment through the Arab target group. Eventually, therefore, ITC's trauma management merged with Israel's ethno-national hierarchy.

Attaching trauma to the sociopolitical context exposed the management to mental vulnerability among all players involved: experts, donors, and the potential aid recipients. The identification of the Jewish settlers and the Palestinians as "those in need" remained suspended between medicalization and demedicalization. Concurrently, a context-related transition occurred from the interpretation of trauma as a psychiatric diagnosis to the interpretation of trauma as a shared cultural experience. The experts made efforts to validate the position of both groups as legitimate victims of a clinical syndrome through professional practices such as "gathering data," "reaching out," "mapping needs," and "screening needs." At the same time, though, the experts and donors used their internal knowledge of the cultural meaning attributed to trauma in Israel, and demedicalized the suffering while reconnecting it to the dominant components and symbols associated with the Zionist narrative.

From a political perspective, this new construction of trauma exemplifies how experts created a space in which inequality is reorganized (Breslau, 2004; James, 2004). However, the inequality articulated is not between the West (specifically, the U.S.) and a weak trauma-stricken nation, but lies within the framework of a single nation. Funded by a Jewish organization from abroad, ITC is independent of the Israeli governmental budget and bureaucracy, but it does not operate on behalf of universal rights. Instead, the Jewish national solidarity shapes its aid discourse. Nevertheless, the various players redefine their competing social standpoints through ongoing negotiation, despite their common background. Here the divide is not between international NGOs, external experts, and local residents. Rather, the social inequalities in Israel involve internal political hierarchies (left-wing secular experts versus right-wing National Orthodox Jewish settlers) and national identity (Israeli-Jewish experts versus Palestinian citizens).

The local politics of trauma, thus, started with the Israeli therapists' interpretation of mental distress as a "standard hallmark," becoming a flexible concept that serves various social players and diverse political interests. In the next chapter, this politics of trauma increases in terms of complexity, and it will turn out that not only are trauma experts dealing with the clinical categories of trauma and PTSD but so are the donors, business people, and philanthropists.

Chapter Two

Trauma and Capital: Bearers of Knowledge, Keepers of Cashboxes

From this podium, I would like to send a warm hug to all the residents [of southern Israel] near the Gaza Strip who, during the past seven years, have not known any peace ... NATAL is dealing and will continue to deal with this [mental aid] challenge and with strengthening the residents' resilience ... This tenth-anniversary event has enabled NATAL to raise 1,200,000 [Israeli shekels] ... I would personally like to thank Nochi Dankner, chairman of the IDB Group and the chief sponsor of the event; and thanks also to Klal Insurance, Dan Hotels, Cellcom, Ashdar, Caraso and Bank Hapoalim.[1]

> – Yehudit Yovel-Recanati, speaking at the tenth-anniversary event for NATAL, 29 February 2008

The first chapter described the political dynamic around trauma as arising from the tension between the clinical concerns of the therapists and the local circumstances of its application. However, the above remarks made by Yehudit Yovel-Recanati, the founder and chair of NATAL, reveal that, in shaping the meaning of both the diagnostic concepts and the way they were applied, the therapists had important partners: business people and philanthropists. Tense relations developed in Israel between the state agencies and non-governmental organizations (Shamir, 2008; Silber, 2008), such as NATAL and ITC. These non-governmental agencies, unlike the state agencies, operated with

---

1 All of these are large companies that have been operating in the Israeli market for the last few decades.

almost no governmental financial support, thus depending almost exclusively on donations. While NATAL received donations from within Israel, especially from the Yovel-Recanati family, the ITC relied on the financial support of the UJA-Federation.

This intriguing partnership is a local manifestation of a broader socioeconomic change in Israeli society and the Western world. Accelerated privatization in Western societies in recent decades (Adams, Van Hattum, and English, 2009; Rhodes, 1996) paved the way for the appearance of "new philanthropy" (Bornstein, 2009; Elisha, 2008). Unlike the old one, what characterizes the new philanthropy is the emergence of donors from their passive stance, transforming them into "donor-entrepreneurs" (Silber, 2008). They stand behind the establishment of new NGOs, and through that become involved in shaping agendas and decision-making processes. The professional support granted by NATAL to the residents of southern Israel was an example of this transformation. It may have been therapeutic support by its very essence, but it was made possible in actuality by virtue of the 1,200,000 Israeli shekels collected from wealthy families like the Dankners and from successful companies like Klal Insurance and Ashdar.

In this chapter, I shed light on the connection between professional knowledge and capital as they relate to security-based trauma. In particular, I describe how the professional treatment of PTSD has entangled itself with socio-economic power struggles. The first expression of this new social action will be the attempt to bridge the gap between two contradictory meanings: the negative associations identified with traumatic injury (the one of pain, distress, and social marginalization) with the positive associations identified with philanthropy and comfortable access to social and financial resources. Yovel-Recanati, and the unique path of action she set out for NATAL in Israeli society, provided an interesting illustration of how someone attempted to bridge the gap. A second expression of the new connection between professional knowledge and capital is the negotiation over the allocation of resources, and the need to garner empathy and compassion for the disempowered populations in Israel. In light of the changing circumstances of the Arab–Israeli conflict, on the one hand, and internal organizational changes within the philanthropic aid agencies themselves, on the other hand, I show how ITC's therapists and donors had a tense dialogue regarding a series of questions: What portion of resources should be allocated for each population and for what types of distress? Which form of aid should receive funding? And for how long?

Between Two Worlds: Addressing Qassam Rockets while Eating Quinoa Salad with Red Grapefruit

Yehudit Yovel-Recanati was the main figure to whom psychiatrist Dr. Yossi Hadar (who later died of leukemia) turned when he came up with the idea of establishing a non-governmental aid agency for trauma victims of the Arab–Israeli conflict. Yovel-Recanati was known as an experienced therapist and had been a student of Hadar's at one of Israel's universities. However, Hadar also turned to her because she belonged to one of the wealthiest families in Israel. The Recanati family immigrated to Palestine from Greece in the early 1930s and, together with the Caraso family, founded Discount Bank, which grew into the corporation known today as IDB Holdings. In the late 1990s, the Recanati family sold the business to the Dankner family for a sum estimated by the local media to be in the hundreds of millions of dollars. Like many of those involved in philanthropy (Bornstein, 2009; Elisha, 2008; Silber, 2008), in interviews she granted to the Israeli media and to me, Yovel-Recanati offered a personal explanation for donating funds from her family – both the one she comes from and the one she raised with her spouse, Dr. Israel Yovel (now deceased). She described her desire to continue the long-standing family tradition of contributing to the Israeli community, but for a purpose that she herself marked as important: granting subsidized therapeutic aid, independent of the state's institutions with their bureaucratic procedures, to anyone and everyone who has suffered mental injury stemming from the Arab–Israeli conflict.

All these biographical details might have remained in the background of NATAL's activities if Hadar had not died suddenly, leaving Yovel-Recanati alone in the leadership position. Consequently, Yovel-Recanati's way of acting and decision-making became critical to the consolidation of NATAL as a non-governmental aid agency in Israel. "[Yehudit's connections are] very, very significant," explains one of the NGO former managers. "So the moment you enlist the [Israeli] elite, it's a lever ... There are a lot of NGOs – they've got problems, let's say, of reaching all sorts of power sources, and of getting all sorts of things for free, and we've been spared that" (Interview, 4 May 2005).

Yovel-Recanati has never tried to deny the unique connection that her figure represents as an integral part of the economic and social elite of Israel and as a trained therapist, who as such is intimately familiar with the suffering of trauma victims. Right from the beginning, she constructed a course of action that sought to bestow the abundance and glamour of the upper class upon the dark and straitjacketed world of the trauma victims. Various channels of popular culture were the primary means she used for that purpose. "In 1999 Yehudit mounted an event at Hechal Hatarbut [Shrine of Culture – a Tel Aviv concert-hall]," recalled the former manager. "I think that already then she put on a grand show of power" (Interview, 4 May 2005).

Other evenings followed that one. In December 2000, Yehudit sponsored "Open Evening" in an auditorium in central Israel, under the title of "Life in the Shadow of Events," with the participation of one of Israel's popular female vocalists. In January 2002, NATAL produced a CD, *There Is Yet Hope*, with noted recording artists. In June 2003, a leading Israeli news broadcaster hosted a large charity event.

The public event with which this chapter opened – NATAL's tenth-anniversary celebrations – perfectly exemplifies the attempt to bridge the gap between the sociocultural world of the donors and that of trauma victims. Hundreds of invitees gathered in one of the large halls in the popular entertainment district at the Tel Aviv Port on a Friday afternoon in February 2008. Some of the invitees were therapists and administrators from NATAL, but most were business people and members of wealthy families in Israel. Inside the dim hall, there were large windows looking out to the sea, covered with heavy curtains, and tall vases filled with long-stemmed flowers were in every corner. The event opened with a brunch: alcoholic drinks, tomato and mushroom soup, quinoa salad and red grapefruit, roasted chicken with peanuts – all of this bounty was laid out on the large tables or served from stylish platters by well-trained uniformed waiters.

About an hour later, the attention of the hundreds of invitees was drawn to the capacious stage. This part of the event opened with a dance performed by one of the famous dance troupes of Israel. Afterwards, three gigantic semi-transparent screens were set up on stage. Images of terror events, as depicted in the local media, were projected onto the screens. Behind each screen stood a figure reciting a passage from a story concerning some dramatic event in the context of the conflict: the experience of a soldier diagnosed with post-traumatic symptoms in the wake of the 1973 War, the loss of comrades-in-arms during the Second Lebanon War, and exposure to a terror attack on a bus in Jerusalem. The three stories were intermingled, one figure saying something, another continuing, then all three figures tore away the screens behind which they were standing and faced the audience. Their faces were brightly lit, and in unison they asked permission "not to hide anymore." Up to the stage came a leading Israeli news broadcaster who had donated her services on behalf of the NGO for the third time. With another round of rocket fire currently taking place in southern Israel, the broadcaster referred to a photograph of two frightened children, a brother and sister, huddled in the opening of a shipping container. The photograph depicted the little girl trying to comfort her brother after a Qassam rocket wounded him in the arm. "There is nothing like these days to tell how important NATAL is," said the broadcaster. Then she proceeded to describe the audience to which she was speaking:

> There are two circles here today: The first circle is the professional staff that carries the therapeutic mission upon their shoulders. In the second circle are the members of the business community and donors who lend support: financial, emotional, and moral. Between these two circles lies the centre, the connecting heart, the heart of one woman: Yehudit Yovel-Recanati. (29 February 2008, Field Notes)

The broadcaster's remarks, and those spoken immediately afterwards by Yovel-Recanati (cited in part at the beginning of this chapter), demonstrate how a new social network of business people and media figures had organized itself around trauma. Within this network, the handling of the disorder took on a new character. This new character had an impressive force and was saturated with emotion. It was far from the clinic and not necessarily connected to the therapeutic concerns that underlay the professional work. The attempt to garner empathy and financial assistance for mental treatment via such means as music, dance, and media personalities was what stood at the centre. The broadcaster, for example, was willing to lend her familiar face and voice to emphasize the importance of NATAL to Israeli society and attest to the importance of the two groups mingling in the hall, therapists on one hand and business people and donors on the other. Yovel-Recanati, in her remarks, sought to emphasize the mental distress of large civilian populations in Southern Israel and NATAL's commitment to helping them. At the same time, Yovel-Recanati too did not fail to emphasize the important role of the donors and commercial corporations in making it possible to provide mental aid to all those populations.

The development of reciprocal relations with donors and media figures aroused some uneasy feelings among the therapists. For example, when I asked a senior therapist from NATAL about the fundraising events, he said:

From my point of view, there were [in the beginning] excessively large gaps between the outside and the inside, between what could be seen from the outside and the content there was inside [NATAL]. In the first stage of NATAL's professional work, there was very little content inside, but to the outside, we looked very, very big. And these gaps were a little dissonant to me. (Interview, 24 July 2005)

The disparity between the "big" representation of trauma directed outward and the "small" mental drama experienced inside the clinic was also reflected in remarks by a young therapist from NATAL's community team. During an interview, the therapist referred to the fundraising event at Hechal Hatarbut in Tel Aviv a few days earlier. She described the event as, "Very large, very present in a certain social consciousness." Then she expressed her reservations, explaining, "It doesn't necessarily make the basic work different." She described a therapeutic intervention that she had been part of several days prior to the fundraising event:

We drove to Beer Sheva [in southern Israel] to work with police officers, in some crowded room; there were very angry people and the air conditioning was hardly working … From my point of view, there is a gap between something in NATAL that is kind of very "social," a lot of social consciousness, and the society itself which in many places is very – it's very small, it's very small, versus the size of this event. There is something very small in the person that you meet, very modest, very – these kinds of shacks, you know, versus all this glamour and glory. (Interview, 2 July 2005)

The therapist, as can be seen, emphasized the great distance, both actual and symbolic, between the participants at the fundraising event and those who had experienced traumatic injury. Donors and representatives of business companies versus police officers, the Shrine of Culture in Tel Aviv versus a crowded room with ineffective air conditioning in Beer Sheva, the glamour of the fundraising event versus the modest, and sometimes the wretchedness that accompanies the therapeutic intervention itself.

That unease was not confined merely to rhetorical protest. In an attempt to resolve the muddle arising before their eyes between clinical concerns and the need to raise funds, over the years NATAL senior therapists drew up working procedures that excluded the administrators, even Yovel-Recanati, from the decision-making process. Michal

Amitai-Tehori, NATAL executive head from 2001 to 2006, candidly revealed the existence of that process:

> Here, there is somehow a very powerful struggle between the professionals and those who aren't professionals. In fact it's a struggle that was born historically at the start of the road, ironically enough, against Yehudit, who is herself a therapist. They couldn't stand that she functioned in two capacities, that she was also the chairwoman, but on the other hand, she used to sit in on the meetings of the professionals ... It was a festering wound that used to burst each time in this context. The kind of anger they used to feel, as if the non-professionals were interfering where only the professionals should, in this sort of "professional temple." (Interview, 4 May 2005)

Amitai-Tehori's remarks demonstrated the "boundary work" (Gieryn, 1999) that the NGO senior therapists were doing in front of Yovel-Recanati. The senior therapists sought to set limits against the immense power they felt she held based on her holding a significant financial capital. This attempt was based especially on their symbolic capital, their professional knowledge and expertise, when NATAL's senior experts have refused to allow her to participate in professional meetings. This boundary work is especially interesting in light of the fact that Yovel-Recanati, as Amitai-Tehori mentioned, is a therapist. Ostensibly, there was really no reason not to allow her to attend those meetings. However, from the senior therapists' point of view, her financial capital was what defined her place in the NGO as the founder and chair. Therefore, it preempted her professional knowledge, and her presence at the professional meetings led to the complaint that "the non-professionals were interfering where only the professionals should." In a personal conversation that took place long afterwards, Yovel-Recanati said to me:

> When the request came up to separate my place from the clinical side, it was difficult for me, but I accepted it. I had to relinquish my involvement in the clinical side, so that NATAL would operate in a clean and professional fashion – free of considerations irrelevant to treatment. This was a decision that ultimately was correct. (Interview, 12 May 2013)

"There may be changes in priorities": Negotiating Financial Resources

Alongside the attempt to use popular culture to bridge the gap between the philanthropists and the trauma victims, an intriguing new interdependency arose between the therapists and the donors. This interdependency revolved around the constant negotiation regarding the type of therapeutic interventions and the allocation of financial resources, often for the sake of organizational survival. However, a soft gentle glow characterized this negotiation within NATAL, thanks to the local familial philanthropy and the warm relations between Yovel-Recanati and the NGO senior professional staff. In contrast, the negotiation in ITC was much harsher. The UJA-Federation stood behind the establishment of ITC, and over the years has been one of its primary donors. Thus, unlike most of the anthropological research about the implementation of the trauma discourse, which focuses on Western humanitarian organizations providing mental aid to residents of non-Western countries (Breslau, 2004; Dwyer and Santikarma, 2007; James, 2004), here the donors held a dual position as social players. The UJA-Federation shared both a historical background and common religious roots not only with the trauma experts but also with the subjects of aid: the Jewish residents of Israel. At the same time, they were separated by both geopolitical and cultural boundaries. Therefore, vibrant negotiation took place in ITC, which has typified its activity and become an unfailing source of misgivings, misunderstandings, and frustrations.

The core of these negotiations lay in a series of guiding principles that were determined shortly after the establishment of ITC in order to regulate the work of the NGOs that joined as members of the new enterprise. These principles attest to the high level of monitoring required of the therapeutic professionals by the donors. The psychologists and psychiatrists at the head of each of the target groups established within ITC were required to provide the donors with comprehensive details regarding the type of intervention they intended to perform using the donated funds. Examples of comprehensive details required on the request forms for funding included the following: target population for intervention, type of intervention, professional service providers, location of the project and its geographic distribution, identification and characterization of recipients' needs, number of aid recipients, identification and characterization of the service providers' needs. Donors made it clear to the heads of all the target groups that there would also be ongoing monitoring of the quality of the intervention and its efficiency, usually by dividing it into several stages and conditioning the performance of each stage on the donor's satisfaction with the previous stage's degree of success.

This constant monitoring intensified in October 2006. A young Jewish attorney from Australia residing in Israel joined the ITC council. Her job, as explained to the therapists at one of the council meetings, was to send bimonthly reports to the UJA-Federation's representatives in New York on the ongoing activity of the target groups. For that purpose, the attorney requested that the therapists submit to her numerical data and qualitative reports to clarify "what's happening, what's being done, where problems are appearing, while gathering information from various sources" (22 October 2006, Field Notes). All of the NGO's representatives expressed their outrage over the new working procedure. One of the psychologists vehemently protested:

> PSYCHOLOGIST: I wasn't trained for this nor is it my job!
> ANOTHER PSYCHIATRIST (in reference to the tracking forms the attorney had distributed): How is it possible to contend with all these items?
> ITC CEO (answering both of them): You can decide [if] it's impossible to cope with it, but we're being told that it would be a mistake in fundraising and in consciousness. [The goal is] to highlight something else every two weeks.

The tense relations between ITC therapists and Jewish-American donors must be understood in light of the starting point of their relationship. From the beginning, the UJA-Federation limited its commitment to funding the activities of ITC for only three years. In an interview, the UJA-Federation representative in Israel explained this limitation: "There is awareness that traumatic injury is long-standing," she said, but then went on to add:

> In New York, there is interest also in other topics, for example poverty in Israel, and the need for developing employment programs. We are not going to stay with trauma and that's it, and there may be changes in priorities ... The donors may be more attentive to this or that field. There are sometimes topics that arise because of current events, poverty, and the Intifada. And there are the donors' plans. (Interview, 19 March 2006)

The termination of funding by the philanthropic body to the agency providing aid generated considerable uncertainty. This translated into two levels of negotiation. On the one hand, ITC therapists attempted to represent the local distress before various philanthropic bodies, in order to sustain ongoing financial resources concurrent with preserving their professional autonomy. On the other hand, there were deliberations among the various NGO members of the ITC about how the local distress should be presented to the donors, as well as how funds were to be distributed among the therapists.

Between Therapists and Donors: "You have to be sexy"

Danny Weitzman, an ITC senior psychiatrist, bitingly described the complex relations that developed between the therapists and the Jewish-American donors. Despite the fact that he was affiliated with a hospital, which might at times seek donations but was not dependent on them for its existence, he depicted the intersection between the professional treatment of trauma and socio-economic power struggles as follows:

> It's clear that the master of the purse strings has the last word ... The moment they approve the budgets and the projects, then certainly they dictate ... By the very fact that [they] approve certain projects and not others, a reality is created ... [The donors] had an agenda of their own that may have suited some members of ITC, and may not have suited others. (Interview, 9 April 2006)

These remarks clearly reflect one of the implications of the "new philanthropic" (Silber, 2008; Shamir, 2008): how the power in the decision-making process changed hands from the therapists to the donors. The donors' personal wishes and subjective impressions strongly influenced their authority to make decisions regarding aid interventions.

ITC council meetings repeatedly gave expression to this tangled intersection of clinical questions and the donors' perspective. For example, at a meeting that took place in December 2005, it emerged that it was entirely unclear whether the UJA-Federation intended to continue supporting ITC in the future. Right at the start of the meeting, an ITC manager, Nurit Ne'eman, shared the following information with the participants:

> NURIT NE'EMAN: On Wednesday, I had a conference call with Lucy, the [Jewish] representative in New York. Lucy began with how proud they are of the ITC. Just the same, she said she was very sorry she didn't get back to me on the matter of ITC's continuation. It appears to be that [one of the managers there] whose interest is in trauma is leaving her position, and it is being transferred to [someone else] who is more interested in poverty. The conclusion was that [out of] the allocated resources ... they are thinking of allocating $150,000 to the entire topic of trauma, and

they haven't yet decided how to give the money. Just the same, they're suggesting that ITC should join the "Capital Campaign," an [overall] fundraising drive ... ITC has to agree on priorities, whether to talk only about trauma, or to also consider poverty and the elderly.

DR. LIORA SHANI (clinical psychologist from one of the NGOs, who had also taken part in the call with UJA-Federation's representatives): The "Capital Campaign" is a multi-annual conception, what you want things to look like in general, and [then get] support for a period of years ... [There are many candidates] ... and you have to be sexy.

NURIT NE'EMAN (ADMINISTRATOR, explaining that one of the UJA-Federation's representatives had provided an example): The elderly with previous traumas, contending with advanced age. It's a topic that can be integrated.

VERED GAL (CLINICAL PSYCHOLOGIST FROM ONE OF THE NGOS): The deep pockets of [the donors in New York] don't exist anymore.

DR. HAIM KATZ (PSYCHIATRIST): Until the next [terror attack on a] building, until the next war. (19 December 2005, Field Notes)

The above exchange demonstrates how an internal organizational change among the donors had the potential to make a dramatic change in the ITC agenda. When one donor left her position to be replaced by another, the focus was no longer on trauma exclusively in the context of the Arab–Israeli conflict, but had shifted to focus on two other new contexts, those of poverty and the elderly. Furthermore, this organizational change led to a reduction in the allocation of resources: the $150,000 pledged to ITC was a much lower sum than it had previously received. The invitation to participate in a fundraising drive was the practical and symbolic expression of these changes. The therapists needed to move from the position of recipients to the position of yielders of proceeds. In order to gain prominence and have value that justified financial investment, they had no choice but to be "sexy." However, against what might have appeared to be a long-term structural change in relations with the donors, Katz's response exposed the fragility of this new phase as well: the donors' interest in poverty at the expense of trauma would only last "until the next [terror attack on a] building, until the next war."

A few days before the abduction of two IDF soldiers along the Lebanese border in northern Israel and a short while after the abduction of IDF soldier Gilad Shalit by Hamas along the Gaza border in the south, the attempt to stabilize relations with the donors reached an impasse. Inbal Levin, a senior administrator, opened the council meeting by conferring with the staff about a conference call she would have in the next few hours with a representative of the UJA-Federation and asking for input:

> We've attained more than we ever dreamed! ... [But] what's happening [among the donors in New York] – there is a very big change not just in priorities but also in sentiments and in how the work is done. The woman who coordinated the trauma field [at the UJA-Federation] was removed from her job and transferred to a truly clerical position ... She won't be replaced ... This could be a wonderful opportunity, but it also puts things in a more complicated place ... There were complaints about their asking for a \$2-million plan within 15 minutes ... So I'm asking [all of] you: What am I supposed to say? What are we asking for today at six-thirty in the evening, in the conference call? (2 July 2006, Field Notes)

Levin's remarks reveal how the intersection between clinical questions regarding aid intervention and the changing social circumstances became more intense due to the critical dependency on philanthropy. Despite ITC having consolidated its position ("We've attained more than we ever dreamed"), a large question mark remained with regard to its economic strength. Apparently, that doubt translated into a deep instability in the financial negotiation process: prolonged deliberations for months over the implementation of a certain plan, and then suddenly "asking for a \$2-million plan within 15 minutes." Levin's remarks provoked a debate among ITC therapists:

> RUTH SHALEV (CLINICAL PSYCHOLOGIST): All of the NGOs here have an interest in maintaining ITC, and we need to say [to the UJA-Federation representatives] that we're on the brink. You [the administrator] need to say [to the UJA-Federation] that they were the actor that began the entire process of observation of trauma in Israel, and they cannot abandon it now. We need financial support and [economic] backing.
>
> DR. IDO LAHAV (PSYCHIATRIST): Really, the members of ITC, at the expense of their time and energy, are clinging on by their teeth to the knowledge that Israel is in a difficult period. The fire can spread; the city of Ashkelon [in southern Israel] is within range, and all of the nearby localities, and we don't know what's going to happen in the north; and people here, without support, continue to persevere in ITC. And it's the donors' time now to support the topic. This body can either enter its time of flowering or simply die.

DR. HAIM KATZ (PSYCHIATRIST): I don't want to be the poor one asking
for pocket money. ITC is barking and kicking, and [if there aren't any
donations], there won't be a coalition. (2 July 2006, Field Notes)

More than anything else, this dialogue attests to the attempt by ITC
therapists to find their way through the maze into which they had
stumbled. On the one hand, there was an apparent plea for continued
financial support from the Jewish-American donors. This request was
not based merely on a clinical premise, such as the expected cessation
of certain intervention programs due to a lack of funding. Rather, it
was based on a nationalist incident in the face of the abduction of the
IDF soldier in the south, and the forecasts of a violent outbreak in
the north, which indeed occurred. ITC therapists, thus, gave a flavour of
national enterprise to their professional activities. Yet they also sought
to retain a certain measure of professional autonomy and to avoid self-
negation as much as they could. Thus, in order to receive ongoing financial support, the therapists considered various alternatives for presenting the mental distress of civilian populations in the north and
south to the donors. Caught between opposing potential outcomes, a
"time of flowering" versus organizational "death," the therapists creatively sought to maintain the new aid agency they had established.

Therapists among Themselves: "No second-class disaster for me"

The complicated relations that developed between the therapists and
the donors gave rise to heated debates among the therapists themselves, who negotiated over the visibility of the traumatic injury that
each of them sought to advance before the donors in order to ensure
prominence for their professional work. At the core of the negotiations
stood the award of "seniority" status to trauma in the context of the
Arab–Israeli conflict and the relegation to secondary status, if any, to
traumatic injuries sustained in other circumstances. The representative
of the Israel Crisis Management Center (ICMC), for example, an NGO
established to deal with immigrants' distress, described the significance
of this process in her interview:

On the first day in ITC, I said several things. One of them was that you are
PTSD of a national background, but for me there is no second-class disaster
and no first-class disaster ... At the time of the [Second] Intifada, when the
funds were intended for [traumatic injuries stemming from] terrorism, I

said that I'm sitting here for one reason: to make sure that others who suffer losses [as a result of other causes than the conflict] will also receive the aid ... There is no reason to differentiate between terrorism and not terrorism. Look, there is cause to differentiate, but there is nothing to compare, all suffering is suffering. (Interview, 8 May 2006)

However, even the creation of an initial hierarchy among various forms of mental distress did not lead to agreement, but gave rise to new debates. As anthropologists have argued (Breslau, 2004; Fassin and Rechtman, 2009), the traditional approach in trauma therapy is directed at the individual. However, during the last two decades, the professional focus has turned mainly to large group intervention, and ITC adopted this new trend. The decision to allocate financial and organizational resources to support such interventions pushed aside individual clinical treatment of post-trauma victims. Later in her interview, the ICMC representative said that during ITC council meetings she invested considerable effort so that "the direct services to the individual in distress [would be] at the forefront of the struggle. Someone has to be there for the individual" (Interview, 8 May 2006).

This debate was far from purely professional. The battle over the ITC agenda clearly carried economic significance. Drawing up therapeutic intervention plans of one kind or another and submitting them for funding by donors affected each of the NGOs' scope of activity and, correspondingly, the size of the financial allocation their people would receive. One prominent example was the gap between the allocations of financial resources to children in comparison to the elderly. For example, at a council meeting held in September 2006, a clinical psychologist from one of the NGOs argued: "There's a feeling that children will receive a lot of money from ITC, and other projects won't." Dr. Katz, a psychiatrist from one of the hospitals, elaborated on this argument:

I'm afraid there are two to three very active target groups, and all the funds will go in that direction. I'm not begrudging them, but when all the budgets arrive, we should have some oversight as to how the budgets will be distributed. (10 September 2006, Field Notes)

This exchange sheds light on how the therapists and the donors turned into "brokers of trauma" (James, 2004). They became the "gatekeepers" who determined which kinds of suffering ought to be helped, who could provide aid, how, and at what cost. For example, the representative of one of the NGOs, which dealt extensively with treatment of the elderly, pointed out "how hard it is to bring up the aging population as a topic ... the treatment of post-traumatic elderly" (interview, 9 April 2006). Within ITC, some explained this gap between the elderly and children as being a result of the children's "power of attraction" for the donors. Naturally, children are a representation of "the pure victim" (Malkki, 1996), thus easily able to cross the physical and cultural boundaries between donors and aid receivers and push aside complex issues such as policy and politics. For that reason, some of the therapists asserted, it was possible to garner recognition, empathy, and resources on behalf of children's distress as opposed to the mental distress of the elderly.

Conclusion

The establishment of NATAL and ITC as active NGOs dependent on the ongoing financial support of donors placed the politics that developed around trauma and PTSD not only at the core of the negotiations among the therapists but also inside their tense interactions with their philanthropic sources. Against the background of the state's withdrawal from its traditional commitments (Adams, Van Hattum, and English, 2009; Rhodes, 1996; Shamir, 2008), Israeli and other philanthropic agencies have played a crucial part in defining the professional approach to security-based trauma management.

Both Yovel-Recanati and the UJA-Federation created new requirements for long-term, subsidized mental aid, independent of Israel's moral and bureaucratic logic. This modus operandi released funding for mental aid from the state's monopoly. However, it also imposed stipulations on what qualified as "suffering," and thus as a legitimate object of aid. Consequently, clinical issues were inseparably linked to socio-economic issues and in the face of that, a need arose not only to treat mental distress but also to represent it. There was a necessity to translate mental distress into channels of popular culture in order to represent it in a "sexy" and exciting way, thus ensuring economic and organizational strength.

However, this dynamic captured in part the significance of the new civic platform for funding mental aid. The operation of the two NGOs indicates how trauma management required the development of a new "moral sensitivity" (Shamir, 2008): the effort to create heightened alertness to mental injuries in the context of prolonged and controversial political conflict in an age of increasing privatization and a decline in collectivist values in Israel (Bilu and Witztum, 2000). The local ramifications of the politics surrounding trauma resulted in an attempt to arrive at an agreed prioritization of the mental suffering that would be acceptable to the various social players from diverse socio-economic and ideological backgrounds. Indeed, these negotiations over social recognition and financial resources were fraught with inherent conflict. Yet this process was necessary in order to fill the financial gap left by the privatized state – "because it's not there, because the state isn't giving it," as one of ITC's psychologists said.

The next chapter deals with an additional intersection that evolved within the new politics surrounding trauma. This time, it was between the very private experience of mental distress and the mass media.

Chapter Three

Trauma and the Camera:
Labelling Stress, Marketing the Fear

There's nothing we can do, in the age of mass communication in which we live, in order to excite, in order to make people identify, feel a connection, you have to put out stories ... And with all due respect, if I bring along a seventy-year-old person who was injured in a terror attack – not that I'm putting it down – it just doesn't work! Because there's nothing to be done. The world belongs to the young ... And you have to bring along men too. There can't be only women, and he can't talk only about terror attacks. He has to talk about shellshock as well – about the traumas that occurred in the course of his military service – and they really don't want it to be someone from the 1973 War, but someone from [a military operation in recent years in the Gaza Strip, for example], or let's say from [an operation that took place in Lebanon].
– Senior marketing manager, NATAL, 26 April 2005

The above remarks by a NATAL senior marketing manager clearly indicate how the politics swirling around trauma in Israel expanded into a new arena: public relations. It turned out that the tension between the clinical concerns and the particular social circumstances of their local application was no longer between therapists and donors but had extended to the social dynamics surrounding labelling, representation, and marketing. The high dependency on donations (see chapter 2) necessarily required the representation of the mental distress in the public sphere, thereby achieving visibility and drawing financial resources. From that inevitable process sprang a hierarchy created by a NATAL senior marketing manager. This hierarchy differentiated between victims of trauma and between the levels of compassion each victim aroused. Basically, the marketing manager constructed a map, not for the treatment of the disorder but for selling it. Accordingly, it was important to represent trauma through the personal story of the victim. For example, it could be a young one, because "the world belongs to the young." Alternatively, it could be about a man who had sustained a mental injury from a war, but not from a terror attack. However, it could not be from an "old" war like the 1973 War, but needed to be from a "new" war like the one in the Gaza Strip or in Lebanon.

This chapter deals with this intense effort to label the distress and to market the fear, and traces the new representation of those emotions in the Israeli media. The representation and distribution of suffering to target audiences around the globe had already been acknowledged as one of the most intricate issues in the era of mass communication (see Boltanski, 1999). However, whereas this task has been much discussed as taking place within the context of Western countries that grant humanitarian aid to non-Western countries, in the Israeli case, this activity has been held within one national context. Humanitarian activists insist on representing the suffering of non-Western populations in disaster or conflict areas in order to overcome the barriers of physical and cultural distance. In Israel, mental distress has relied on a sense of shared belonging within a single national community and based on a familiarity with one political conflict. For precisely these reasons, I show how the presentation of mental suffering demanded a high degree of improvization, creativity, and sensitivity. The experts, together with the marketing advisers, searched for new and effective presentations of the mental suffering while addressing various target groups. Furthermore, they used – and avoided from using – particular cultural content in order to leverage certain narratives of trauma and forms of coping among Israeli and North American audiences.

In what follows, I present the change in NATAL's name and logo related to three languages (Hebrew, English, and Arabic) and two visual icons: the flag and the tree. In addition, I describe how therapists, together with the public relations team, sought to market trauma through the production of the film *Wounded in Soul*. In the shooting of the film, the way in which three authentic stories of trauma were narrated before the camera while using several artificial techniques reveals how the narrators were turned into "talents of trauma."

The Name and Logo: Different Meanings in Hebrew, English, and Arabic

At the beginning of 2001, three years after NATAL was established, its founders sought to examine the Israeli attitude towards the NGO's activities. The purpose of the inquiry was not to evaluate the position of potential users with regard to the aid services but to explore the NGO's public image among "the established middle class" (Research Report, 2001, Field Notes). Four focus groups of Israeli citizens ages twenty to sixty, all of them identified with the upper-middle class, were convened for the purpose of ascertaining the participants' attitudes towards the NGO's name at the time, which was the Center for Mental and Social Aid for Trauma Victims of a National Background. Another focus group consisted of "people of an Anglo-Saxon mentality, who represented potential donors" (Research Report, 2001, Field Notes). The researchers' main conclusion from the focus groups was that the NGO's public image was quite problematic. Paradoxically, the problem lay in the primary object of its activity as represented by the keyword in its name: trauma.

> Most of the participants thought that "the criterion of trauma" did not provide the people who were in a situation of stress or dysfunction as a result of the security situation in Israel a legitimate reason for turning [to NATAL]. (For example, those who don't go out to malls or are afraid to send their children to school or worried for their sons serving in the army.) (Research Report, 2001, Field Notes)

In light of this finding, the researchers recommended changing the NGO's name to Center for Aid in Situations of Stress and Trauma of a National Background.[1] They explained that the two new keywords added to the NGO's name, "stress" and "situation," would make it possible to educate the public about the possibility of receiving aid in relatively "mild" stress situations. In addition, these terms would deliver the message that the NGO "devotes itself to assisting a broad population that has been injured to some degree from a national-security event" (Research Report, 2001, Field Notes). As can be seen, this reasoning integrates the clinical concerns regarding trauma treatment with social issues. The term "stress" portends a world of content consisting of difficulties much more normative and mundane than trauma. Furthermore, the term "situation" makes it possible to disconnect the

---

1 A few years later, following a strategic program conducted by NATAL, the NGO's name was changed again. At that point, the term "stress" was eliminated and the name became "Trauma Victims of a National Background."

experience of distress and trauma from a particular personality type that might be identified with pathology, and to connect the mental difficulties to everyday life in Israel. Therefore, these two indicators, "stress" and "situation," make it possible to wrap the mental injury in a much friendlier package than the initial version, and NATAL senior staff immediately adopted both versions.

Another recommendation by the research team was rejected. The focus group findings revealed that just like "trauma," the keyword "national" in the NGO's name was perceived as problematic. The researchers reported that most of the participants were convinced the name created identification between the NGO and the Jewish people in Israel. Some of the participants even asserted that the NGO should also be given a name in Arabic, "to encourage Arab–Israeli citizens to turn to NATAL too" and "to communicate that this is a pluralistic and liberal organization" (Research Report, 2001, Field Notes). Nonetheless, the NGO's senior staff left the keyword "national" in place. Although the experts broadened their aid to include a vast array of mental experiences, from simple fear to severe post-traumatic symptoms, they still adhered to one very narrow domain: all the mental conditions had to originate from national conflict. Even NATAL's name in Arabic remained as it was, merely an acronym with no detailed wording.

However, one change in the "pluralistic and liberal" direction was made. The first logo NATAL senior staff used to represent their work visually was one of Israel's "key symbols" (Ortner, 1973): the flag. The name of the NGO was represented in the middle between two lines of blue and white. Yet, just as the focus group had expressed unease regarding the keyword "national," the researchers found that "the present logo is perceived as problematic … It is perceived as worn and too much affiliated with the state, Jewish in a way that is liable to deter the Arab citizens from applying, and arousing an immediate association with the political right wing" (Research Report, 2010, Field Notes). In place of the flag, the researchers proposed the tree, an icon that the focus group perceived as "universal and humane." The NGO adopted this recommendation, and its revised name came to appear beneath the spreading branches of a tree.

The transition from the symbolic marker of a flag to a tree represented new social qualities that NATAL's senior staff asked to identify with the mental condition of trauma: fluidity, ambiguity, and flexibility. The professional "standard" under which the NGO started out was marked by the distinct national icon of the flag and conveyed, as a result, an

unequivocal visual message: mental assistance was for those who suffered from violent conflict between Jews and Arabs. The new icon, the
tree, might be interpreted in varying ways. On the one hand, the tree
relates to the world of nature and, thus, people perceived it as universal
and panhuman. Citing the data from the focus groups, the researchers
noted this. On the other hand, the tree also represents the ideal of oc-
cupying the land and planting roots, a practice identified with a Zionist
nation-building project (Kimmerling, 1993). Still, the tree was a softer
and gentler image than the flag was.

Alongside the Hebrew representation, the researchers also looked
into the name of the NGO in English. Perhaps contrary to expectations,
NATAL's name in English was not a direct translation of its name in
Hebrew, and included slightly different keywords: the Israel Support
Center for Victims of National Psychotrauma. The difference between
the names in the two languages indicates that NATAL senior staff assumed they were addressing two different target audiences. With these
different names, they "packaged" the professional treatment of trauma
differently on behalf of each audience. However, the NGO's English
name, just like the Hebrew name, did not pass the focus group test. In
the wake of the participants' responses, the researchers insisted that the
name in English was problematic:

> Too long, unclear, not focused enough, and it doesn't clarify what the or-
> ganization really is. [It would be preferable to use] strong words, charged
> and clear, such as "war" and "terror," "victims," "trauma," each of which
> has a powerful emotional resonance and conjures an entire world of as-
> sociations concerning Israel. (Research Report, 2001, Field Notes)

The NGO's name in English was indeed changed to Israel Trauma
Center for Victims of Terror and War. The difference between the name
in English and the name in Hebrew, Center for Aid in Situations of
Stress and Trauma of a National Background, attests to the nature of the
distinction drawn by NATAL senior staff between Hebrew speakers
and English speakers. In addressing the local Jewish-Israeli target audience, NATAL sought to establish mental distress as an identity-shaping
experience bound up with daily life in Israel. Therefore, they deliberately
avoided limiting the distress to specific causes and hoped to encourage the seeking of aid for a wide range of mental injuries. Conversely,
in addressing the audience outside Israel, especially North American
Jews, the cord that tied trauma to the national context of Israel was

severed and replaced by one that tied the disorder to "terror" and "war." This packaging sought to give trauma a more global quality by emphasizing elements that people would perceive as causing mental suffering all over the world, certainly after the events of September 11. Therefore, NATAL chose to express the suffering through an already well-known, highly legitimate status in the West: "victims" (Bob, 2002; Fassin, 2008; Malkki, 1996).

Wounded in Soul: Narratives of Trauma between the Authentic and the Artificial

In the summer of 2005, NATAL senior staff reached a decision to produce a film about the NGO's activities that would serve as a fundraising instrument in Israel and abroad. Despite the consensus on the importance of the film, deep tension between the marketing team of NATAL and its therapists accompanied the production process. The marketing team insisted that the actual trauma victims at NATAL had to appear in the film in order to present a link between the mental injury and the aid services offered by the NGO. The therapists, though, refused to approach their patients and propose they take part in the filming. They asserted that such an act could not be reconciled with therapeutic ethics requiring the maintenance of clear boundaries between the clinic and the outside world. However, they were willing to offer themselves as potential participants for the aim of describing the meaning of traumatic injury and the need to receive aid. The marketing team repeatedly rejected that offer, claiming that explanations by therapists, fluent as they may be, could not arouse sufficient emotion, lead to empathy, and prompt philanthropy.

In the end, they reached a compromise. Two patients of NATAL, Zohar and Shai, both in their thirties, had concluded a therapeutic process, and their therapists agreed to make an exception and find out whether they were willing to participate in the film. They both agreed. Sari, a bereaved mother whose son was killed when on duty as a soldier in the Gaza Strip, also offered to play a part in the film. However, Sari had received treatment by the Ministry of Defense and, therefore, did not fit the criteria set by the marketing team: being a patient of NATAL. Yet, in light of the therapists' refusal to approach patients, one of the NGO administrators used her personal connection with Sari to propose she take part in the film. Thus, these were the three primary participants in the film: Zohar, Shai, and Sari.

In September 2005, I joined NATAL's senior marketing manager and the production crew during the filming in the private homes of Zohar, Shai, and Sari. It soon became evident that besides the cameras and sound equipment there was another essential tool: the "Chinese lotion." When the lotion was applied beneath the eyes, it gave the moist appearance of recent tears. Use of the lotion attested to how the filmmakers sought to represent trauma. It became, then, a means of distinguishing between the three participants: To whom would they suggest applying the lotion? To whom wouldn't they? Who would agree, and who would refuse? And who wouldn't need the lotion because his or her tears were real?

Zohar, Mall Security Guard: "I'm stepping on pieces of people!"

The movie's first participant was Zohar, twenty-eight years old, a student, married, and the mother of a baby girl. When a suicide bombing occurred at a mall in central Israel in May 2001, Zohar was working there as a security guard. The terrible sights she saw left an indelible imprint on her memory, disrupting her daily routine and leading to her being diagnosed as suffering from PTSD. That is how she came to receive mental treatment at NATAL. A few months after her treatment concluded, she agreed to take part in the film *Wounded in Soul*. Before the shooting began, the makeup technician suggested that Zohar apply the Chinese lotion under her eyes. Zohar agreed. Then the director asked her to sit on a chair in the kitchen; behind her, at an angle carefully contrived by the photographer, stood the rack for her baby girl's bottles and pacifiers. The shooting began:

DIRECTOR: Let's go back, to the time you were working as a security guard at the Sharon Mall. It was a Friday.
ZOHAR: I arrived at the mall after a college exam to arrange my shifts … Suddenly we heard a pretty serious boom, like a detonation. I felt a powerful shock wave over my body. Right away, we understood it was a terrorist attack. We ran outside. We understood it was what we thought, what we saw …
DIRECTOR: I want you to say "I saw," "I thought" – it's more personal.
ZOHAR: I passed the first pedestrian crossing; there were lots of pieces on the floor, on the road. At the third crossing, I couldn't go on anymore. It was too crowded with pieces. I didn't want to touch them with my

fingers ... [There was] absolute silence, and lots of scattered clothes and bits [of flesh], scattered people ... You saw bones, how white they were. I pressed forward. There were the spilled guts of a human being. There was someone's arm ... I called my mother, my boyfriend, Guy. I called my grandmother, to say that everything was all right. I was all right, everything was not all right ... The people who passed by, they had remains of people stuck to them ...

DIRECTOR: Stuck to them? Did any stick to you too?

ZOHAR: Someone from the victim identification unit came up to me and said, "Can't you see that you're stepping on pieces?!" I was stepping on pieces of people! ... It made it hard to run. I wished I had shoes or boots on, that they wouldn't touch my skin, my body, the pieces ...

DIRECTOR: What happened in life afterwards, Zohar?

ZOHAR (pausing, looking down, and speaking quietly): I cried all the time; I wanted to sleep all the time; I would get up tired, all the time I was looking for a place to lay my head.

DIRECTOR: And before that, you were alert, active?

ZOHAR: Yes.

DIRECTOR: Did you feel [the change]? Did anyone say anything to you? Couldn't you go home from the college [for example]?

ZOHAR: No, I couldn't. Taking the bus was not an option [because I was afraid of another terrorist attack] ... I didn't want anyone to come see my limbs scattered all over the place! Not to be exposed! I was mad at myself that I was falling apart, that I wasn't in control.

DIRECTOR: What does that mean, not in control?

ZOHAR: I cried all the time, I was unable to let go. I felt that people couldn't stand me ... Riding the bus was so difficult. Where should I sit? Where would he [the terrorist] enter from? Maybe at the back of the bus? But where is the bus's fuel tank? Until the ride would end, it was simply a nightmare. There were also a lot of financial considerations, all along the way, and that's one of the benefits of the place where I received help from. (18 September 2005, Field Notes)

Despite what might have seemed to an outsider observer to be an intense personal disclosure, it turned out that the production crew was dissatisfied. The senior marketing manager asked the director to go back to the nightmares and the decline in Zohar's functioning so she could speak "from a more personal place." The director said, partly jokingly, that Zohar "soaked up all of the Chinese lotion; she makes it disappear!" He then turned to Zohar and tried to explain to her how important it was to describe in detail the mental suffering: "You need to say 'me,' 'me,' 'me,'" he told her. The marketing manager, in support, told her "to bring only yourself. You're not supposed to carry anyone else's flag, not [even] the national flag; you're not in [your country's] service." The filming resumed, and the director asked Zohar to talk about her nightmares.

ZOHAR: It's a twenty-second clip that keeps on returning in a loop; you see it all the time, go into it uncontrollably, like a tape recording. And it starts running and running, and it zooms in on the arm and zooms in on the big piece [of flesh] … It took me time to acknowledge that I needed professional help, someone to help me get it out, because I was liable to lose my sanity.

DIRECTOR: Did life from that moment change? I want you to say it.

ZOHAR (her eyes suddenly filling with tears): My life changed drastically. My life changed entirely; to this day, I haven't gone back to the same routine.

DIRECTOR: Did you think it was radical to seek out [mental] treatment?

ZOHAR: Well, who goes to a psychologist? Nutcases, and I'm not! But at a certain stage I started feeling that I was losing my sanity. And maybe they would be able to get rid of the entire mess. Maybe they would have the patience to listen.

DIRECTOR: How was it in treatment?

ZOHAR: Lifesaving. I couldn't have had a life without it. Slowly, slowly my sanity returned to me.

DIRECTOR: Could you begin the sentence with "The treatment at NATAL gave me my life back"?

ZOHAR: The treatment at NATAL gave me life. It's something that nobody gave me. I didn't get it from the [Israeli] state, that's for sure. No one takes responsibility for these attacks, except for terrorist organizations. And [NATAL] simply saved me … They [at NATAL] considered [treating] me without regard to my payment. If I had [more money], I would have paid much more. It bothered me that I couldn't pay as much as I should have.

DIRECTOR: What's the most amazing thing that happened to you [thanks to the treatment]?

ZOHAR: Since the treatment, I have a life. I have a family. I have my baby girl! I have my baby thanks to NATAL, because during the time, Guy and I separated. It was my therapist who held me together … She helped me believe that he would come back [to me] and we would get married. And that's how it was. I have a life. I've reason to smile.

DIRECTOR (to the marketing team at the end of filming): In the end, we didn't need the lotion; the tears were real. (18 September 2005, Field Notes)

The director's instructions to Zohar, in addition to the makeup and the camera angle, all clearly indicated how the marketing team aspired to represent trauma in the national context of Israel: as dramatic (even melodramatic) a personal narrative as possible. In order to achieve this goal, the director sought to focus on Zohar and her "significant others." The film hinted at the presence of her baby girl, for example, right from the start by seating Zohar at an angle that allowed the camera to capture the rack of bottles and pacifiers in the background. The director also wove in the presence of her partner, Guy. His leaving her and then returning was part of the story of trauma. This focus on Zohar as an individual prepared the second stage for which the production crew was aiming: to represent trauma as the basic dichotomy of life versus death. Therefore, the director concentrated on the dramatic encounter between Zohar's living body and the bodies of the dead in the mall. The corporeal disintegration of the dead and wounded that Zohar described and her fear of the possible disintegration of her own body were presented as an analogy to her mental disintegration: the nightmares, weeping, and dysfunction.

To maintain these boundaries of trauma as an individual and dramatic narrative, the director ignored the socio-economic aspect of Zohar's traumatic injury to which she alluded in describing her need for the treatment to be concluded. Furthermore, Zohar's own criticism of Israel's state agencies, which did not grant enough aid, also received scant attention. "You need to say 'me,' 'me,' 'me,'" the director repeatedly explained to her, while the marketing manager asked her "to bring only yourself." This personal perspective made it possible to represent trauma as a twofold process of transformation: from who Zohar was before the terrorist attack to who she became after it; and from who she was after the attack but before the treatment, to who she became after treatment ("Since the treatment I have a life. I have a family, I have my baby girl"). Despite Zohar's agreement to use the Chinese lotion to give her face the moist appearance of recent tears, ultimately the director measured the success of the reconstruction of her traumatic story by the fact that her tears were real.

Shai, Firefighter: "We were abandoned"

At noontime, we arrived at Shai's home. At thirty-eight years old, Shai was married, a father of three, and working as a firefighter in one of the biggest cities in Israel. In the course of duty, he participated in the evacuation of the dead and wounded from the Park Hotel after a terrorist attack on Passover Eve in March 2002. He hadn't been diagnosed as suffering from PTSD, but various symptoms he reported did relate to the disorder, such as insomnia, nightmares, withdrawal, and angry outbursts that eventually led him to seek therapeutic aid through NATAL's hotline. Before the filming at Shai's home, the director asked him, "How do you feel about crying?" Shai smiled and the director told him about the virtues of the Chinese lotion. He refused. After a series of general questions, Shai began explaining the difficulty he had encountered as a firefighter in a city like Netanya that had suffered numerous terrorist attacks: "One of the major problems [is] that in terms of preparedness for work, we experienced something we hadn't expected." The director interrupted him and requested, "Speak personally: 'me.'" Shai refused, explaining:

> First of all, we function as a collective. I, like most of us, served in the army. I was in a combat unit, but as a citizen, they don't prepare you for this inferno called terrorist attacks. I was at sixteen attacks, including all the big ones … And then came the grand finale at the Park Hotel … We received the call at 19:06. It was a very tense time, Passover Eve. We were getting organized to conduct the Seder dinner. (18 September 2005, Field Notes)

A technical problem interrupted the filming. The director used the break to once again broach the topic of the Chinese lotion with Shai. Smiling, he said to him, "I don't really want [you to cry], but I do want [tears]." Shai relented, and the makeup technician applied the lotion beneath his eyes. Filming resumed with Shai describing what happened in the hotel after the terrorist bombing:

> SHAI: I walk two metres. I see a body on the floor … A killing field that can't be described. Everything topsy-turvy. And then a tidal wave of people that simply overwhelms us. I felt that in another moment I'd fall to the floor. Screaming, reports of the attack begin, and then the real chaos starts; I go inside. Our names appear on our shirts for the sake

of improving the service ... So an elderly woman steps up to me and says, "Listen, Shai, you've got to help me. My husband's inside. Help him. He can't get out." ... I look at him and realize what condition he's in. And she says to me, "Swear to me you'll take care of him." (Bowing his head, weeping silently for a moment) And I say to her, "All right," but it's the living you have to care for, not the dead.

DIRECTOR: That man you saw, her husband – was he dead?

SHAI: Yes, I saw immediately. We start to evacuate people from the hotel pool, [and we had to evacuate] lots of people with wheelchairs. You step into a pool of blood, simple as that, a fish-pool that has turned into a bloodbath.

DIRECTOR: What did you go through [mentally]?

SHAI: At that moment, nothing ... It starts when you get home. And then the bedlam begins. You don't see it at first, don't notice. You do notice but aren't conscious of it. Insomnia sets in at night. You can't sleep, so everything makes you irritable. You have outbursts, and you have young children that are hit by the entire barrage of nerves, and they don't deserve it. Not physically, no blows, but you haven't got patience for anything.

DIRECTOR: Did you have outbursts?

SHAI: Yes. They're listening to the television too loud, and everything bothers you. Food – everything reminds you, flesh, smells. You can't sit down to the table. And those moments when you do get some sleep, it all comes back to you, one more time, and then again, and again and again. (18 September 2005, Field Notes)

At this moment, suddenly, Shai's boys, eight-year-old twins and a two-year-old baby, burst into the room. The production crew welcomed their arrival, and the interview was interrupted to shoot some footage of Shai with his sons. Several minutes later, the children left the room and filming resumed. Glancing at his watch, the director asked Shai to "skip a few stages."

SHAI (smiling, but insistent): It's easy for you to say skip, in the framework of the deception anything goes ... With NATAL I made contact pretty much by accident. The system in Israel doesn't help ... The basis is that you are sent to the army, you are trained to kill in a combat unit. That's what you're channelled and led into ... In my system, people aren't aware of the consequences. I demanded psychological treatment for

myself and for everyone, and you know how the Israelis are – we are
men! We don't need these things [such as mental assistance]! The social
system is collapsing. I don't know how we've fallen so low.

DIRECTOR: Let's stay with Shai.

SHAI: Shai is only part of the story, nonetheless.

DIRECTOR: When did you decide you were wounded?

SHAI: Never. I never thought of it as being wounded, I thought of it as
support and aid ... The contact with NATAL simply stabilized me; put
me back on track. It will never be what it was, and the hoax is a hoax, an
adult person lives in imaginings, lives with the hoax. To laugh with the
children, although inside you're dead, but it's either you throw up your
arms and wither away or you go on, and I went on ... I don't know with
what [resources] this organization called NATAL was established. It's not
governmental. One of the state's crimes is that they send you to fight and
don't take care of you afterwards. We were abandoned, pure and simple.
You keep telling me all the time to say "me," but I have a lot of friends
who are bleeding and unaware of it.

DIRECTOR (after consulting with the photographer): Take a look down.

SHAI (smiling, looking squarely at the camera): It'll be all right.

Unlike Zohar, the filming of Shai exposed a deep tension between how
the participant asked to deliver his traumatic narrative and the one
sought after by the production crew. Shai wanted to tell a group story
of shared experience, and tended to use the plural voice, "we." He referred to the mental injury of the entire group of firefighters he works
with, and pointed the finger of blame at the state for abandoning those
it sent to save lives. Contrary to Zohar, Shai refused to define himself
as "wounded," and he did not attribute any transformative significance to the aid he received from NATAL. Instead, he perceived the aid
as having only a stabilizing quality. However, like Zohar before him,
the production crew wanted Shai to represent his trauma as a personal,
dramatic narrative. Thus, the director asked him to focus on the terrible
events at the Park Hotel, and after that, in his personal life. The difference between how the participant and the director wanted to present
the traumatic narrative gave rise to tension. "It's easy for you to say
skip," Shai rebuked the director, because "in the framework of the hoax,
anything goes." Although Shai acquiesced to using the Chinese lotion,
he refused to lower his head at the end of filming, and instead looked
squarely at the camera and affirmed, "It'll be all right."

Sari, Bereaved Mother: "In one second, the entire world collapsed"

Sari, in her early fifties, lost her nineteen-year-old son Ariel while he was serving as a military photographer in Gaza Strip. Although Sari had received mental aid from the Israel Ministry of Defense rather than NATAL, the marketing team credited great importance to her agreement to participate in the movie. A mother's bereavement over a son fallen during military action is perceived as a distinct manifestation of trauma in the national context of Israel, and that sufficed to push aside the fact that Sari was not NATAL's patient. Furthermore, the way the production crew treated Sari was also very different from the way they treated her co-participants, Zohar and Shai. No one asked Sari to apply the Chinese lotion beneath her eyes; the director gave her hardly any instructions, and spared her leading questions in the course of filming. Sari told her story of losing Ariel in a single take, all of us seated around her:

> SARI: It's a very big hole in the heart, very intense longing, actual physical
>   things: a sort of lump in the throat, eyes that tear up, deprivation, a
>   vacuum, the wish to have just one more minute with him, to feel …
>   Ariel served in the IDF Spokesperson's Office, in Tel Aviv, a non-combat
>   serviceman, and I was at ease. It turned out that he went out a lot to the
>   [Gaza Strip] and didn't tell us … On Sunday, he was supposed to come
>   home, to start a weeklong leave. He called on Saturday that he was going
>   to Beer Sheva [in southern Israel]. At eight in the evening, he called and
>   said, "I've arrived." When he said that, he was already in Rafah. He'd
>   gone into Gaza. We were at a movie theatre with little Itai. We came
>   home and went to bed. At three in the morning, they rang at the gate,
>   and since then our lives have [been] turned upside down. I asked, "Who
>   is it?" He said, "The notification unit." The whole street was full of men
>   in uniform, doctors, escorts, and I still didn't get it. "Ariel was killed in a
>   military operation in Gaza." I said, "That can't be, they've got the wrong
>   house." I still say it today. In one second, our family changed. In one
>   second, the entire world collapsed. At first I would go up to his room a
>   lot, smell him, the shirt he wore before he went down to Gaza. The room
>   is there, but he's not there anymore. You can feel it's an empty room,
>   too tidy … As a mother, I make a great effort to live for Noa [her eldest
>   daughter], for Itai [her younger son], for our family. Though [our family]
>   has changed, it'll manage to survive.

DIRECTOR: You haven't had help from NATAL, right?

SARI: I've had mental help from the Ministry of Defense. You've got to have help, it's impossible to go through it alone. Help in the form of pills, of conversations, of therapy. It's such a big thing that it's impossible to deal with it on your own. You sink. It's like sinking into a swamp. Each day you sink more and more, and you've got to have help and there's no shame in that. (18 September 2005, Field Notes)

The loss of Ariel lent a special quality to Sari's story regarding the presentation of trauma. As opposed to the symbolic or physical existence of Zohar's baby and Shai's children, what was most prominent in Sari's story was Ariel's clear and absolute absence. The incomprehensible gap between the simplicity of the ringing at the gate and the terrible news of loss that it foretold, attested to the immensity of the pain. Ariel's death, his empty room, and Sari's wish to be with him for just another moment, were all expressions of her traumatic injury. The director perceived the finality of the loss as so severe that it alone, without the Chinese lotion and without having received any mental aid from NATAL, sufficed to provide an appropriate presentation of trauma in the national context of Israel. Sari provided a personal story, dramatic and jolting, which was capable of stirring powerful emotions, eliciting empathy, and inspiring donations.

Less than a month after the filming, the movie was screened in front of NATAL's senior staff and marketing team at the production company offices. Everyone in the production crew attended the screening except for the three participants. Since it had been decided that the movie would not be more than ten minutes in length, the three stories underwent extensive editing and were merged to create a three-stage presentation of trauma. In the first stage, the director selected the most dramatic statements from each participant to describe each trauma: Zohar described the blast in the mall and how she found herself stepping on "pieces" of flesh; Shai described the "bloodbath" and the woman who asked him to save her dead husband; and Sari described the ringing at the gate in the middle of the night. In the second stage, the film highlighted the importance of treatment: Sari declared, "You've got to have help"; and Zohar and Shai explained the value of the aid they received from NATAL. In the third and last stage, the focus was on how mental treatment had helped all three participants in their lives after the traumatic event: Zohar explained that treatment had given her back her life and made it possible for her to marry and bear a child; Shai asserted that it put him back "on track"; and Sari just smiled.

The director carefully assembled a mosaic of statements into an overall, concise presentation of mental trauma in the national context of Israel. The power of the presentation lay in the movement, back and forth, between the collective and individual levels. Exposure to Palestinian aggression was wreaking personal mental havoc on the lives of young people and adults and, as a result, was threatening collective harm to one of the central social institutions of Israeli-Jewish society – the family (Herzog, 1999; Moore, 2012; Sachs, Sa'ar, and Aharoni, 2007).

Images of the outcome of these terror attacks in Israel were presented vis-à-vis the three incidents: a young woman present at a terrorist attack in a crowded mall whose mental symptoms almost denied her marriage and motherhood; a young man who evacuated the dead and wounded from a hotel full of celebrants on Passover Eve whose insomnia led to outbursts of rage against his small children; and a mother of three whose middle child was killed in a military operation in the Gaza Strip. The representation of the therapeutic aid as redress for both a personal and social injury complemented the film's transition between the collective and the individual levels. The therapeutic aid Zohar received fortified her to renew the relationship that had been disrupted because of her trauma symptoms, allowing her to give birth to her baby girl and become a mother. The aid Shai received enabled him to get back "on track" and continue fulfilling his role as father in a normative way. Lastly, the aid Sari received allowed her to process the loss of Ariel and serve as a mother to his younger brother and older sister. At the end of the movie's allotted ten minutes, an off-screen narrator declared, "NATAL. We are here to help!"

Conclusion

The change in NATAL's name and logo and the filming of the movie *Wounded in Soul* demonstrated a further extension of the politics that had developed around trauma and PTSD in Israel: from the clinic and professional boardrooms to the arena of labelling and marketing. The handling of the disorder in this new arena did not resonate with clinical questions of diagnosis, treatment, and prevention, nor did it concentrate on issues of professional priorities and the allocation of resources.

Instead, the core of the debate revolved around how to create effective presentations of mental suffering for various target groups. These presentations were developed using – and avoiding – particular cultural content in order to highlight certain narratives of trauma and forms of coping among Israeli and North American audiences.

The challenge of the presentation was even more intense when it confronted not those far from the suffering and distress (Boltanski, 1999), but those familiar with it. In particular, those individuals who did not frame it within the clinical definitions of trauma did not interpret the distress and suffering such that they required therapeutic intervention. Therefore, this challenge raised a series of difficult questions: What was the right way to make a personal narrative public? How should the pain and distress, and with them the therapeutic aid, be conveyed from the personal "inside" to the social "outside"? How should the participants in the film discuss mental distress, not before a psychologist as they usually did, but before movie directors, lighting and makeup technicians? How should loss, shock, nightmares, and anxiety be depicted outside the confines of the treatment room? What is the best way to communicate these personal elements into hundreds and thousands of homes and give a medical title to their distress, thereby encouraging people to undergo therapeutic treatment?

Dealing with these questions of presentation and its moral implications took the negotiations surrounding trauma far beyond the boundaries of the clinical concerns to an almost opposing social rationale, that of mass communication. In contrast to the intimacy of the clinic, the efforts at labelling and marketing have transformed trauma from a distinct clinical concept into "a new way for people to be" (Hacking, 1986: 223). Trauma and PTSD went from being a mental disorder familiar to the select few (the therapists dealing with it) and relevant to a small minority (those diagnosed with it), to a topic with which many people could identify. Furthermore, this attempt to turn diagnostic categories into a familiar experience entailed a tense relationship between the authentic and the artificial. In the end, the changes in NATAL's name and logo did not attest to any essential change in the therapeutic understanding of traumatic injury or in the aid offered by the NGO, nor were they meant to. The addition of the keywords "stress" and "situation" to the NGO's Hebrew name, the replacement of the flag icon with the tree, and the addition of the terms "war" and "terror" instead of "psychotrauma" to the NGO's English name were only a means of relabelling the disorder and the therapeutic work it entailed. These changes sought to achieve visibility, gain prominence, attract donations, and increase use of intervention services.

Similarly, the Chinese lotion, the carefully contrived camera angles, and the director's questions were artificial means of renarrating three authentic stories of trauma. This reconstruction process was perceived as necessary for trauma's "rating" value, which characterizes the era of mass communication. In addition, the director treated the movie's participants, primarily Zohar and Shai, as "presenters" of suffering or "talents" of trauma. What NATAL therapists sought to explain through professional concepts, Zohar, Shai, and Sari presented through their bodies and souls. Like any other "presenter" or "talent," the power of the three lay in their ability to offer a connection between the "I" and the "we." Their personal suffering was an expression of broader suffering, which many Israelis have experienced as a result of the political conflict between Jews and Arabs. Their narratives stood on their own while being interwoven into the collective narrative of the nation. This movement from the personal to the collective made it possible to generate empathy for their suffering yet avoid seeing them as isolated cases in order to demonstrate their public significance.

Although the three participants had experienced emotional dramas and adopted coping strategies that were indeed personal and private, they were presented as embodying relevancy to a large audience: What was the traumatic event that had changed their lives? Might we experience a similar one? How did they cope with it? Will all of us have to deal with it? How had they continued, after struggling and sometimes in the course of it, to live, function and work, to love and raise children, despite the price that the conflict had exacted from them? How should all of us, because of the experiences we have gone through or may still go through, struggle and live, be afraid but continue to love and function?

The following chapters further elaborate on the political dynamic that began to develop among therapists, donors, and the marketing team. The ethnographic gaze turns from the negotiations swirling around trauma within the new organizational platform as discussed in the first three chapters to the professional application of clinical concepts inside, but especially outside, the clinic.

Chapter Four

They Shoot, Cry, and Are Treated: The "Clinical Nucleus" of Trauma among IDF Soldiers

The initial moral engine with which NATAL embarked was the mental distress of combat soldiers of the IDF and repatriated POWs. The NGO's founders felt that the members of these groups had not received enough recognition as potential carriers of trauma, neither from a clinical perspective nor from a public one. Although the outbreak of the Second Intifada swiftly diverted the professional focus onto the trauma of civilians (see Bleich, Gelkopf, and Solomon, 2003; Somer and Bleich, 2005), in September 2005, the pendulum swung back to the target population of IDF soldiers when the NGO launched a new project called "Graduates of the Friction with the Palestinian Population." Professor Bleich, the head of NATAL's steering committee, explained the rationale behind it:

> [It's necessary to reach out to] every Intifada graduate, without necessarily defining the level of distress, so we can give him a platform on which to share his angers, his quandaries ... Our working assumption is that everyone who was there had something done to him. No one remained naïve ... It is a psycho-educational project for society ... It's an educational process of the population. (Steering Committee, 28 September 2005, Field Notes)

As can be seen, the new project served as a means for reframing the meaning of trauma in the context in which it first established its footing: the IDF. As formulated by Bleich, the project reflected NATAL's attempt to break out of the place that, for years, had been allocated for traumatic injuries among soldiers by their colleagues in psychiatric units at the IDF and the Ministry of Defense. The new therapeutic goal as designed by NATAL was for the entire Israeli society to acknowledge every combat soldier who served in the Gaza Strip or the West Bank ("every Intifada graduate, without necessarily defining the level of distress," as Bleich put it) as a potential carrier of trauma.

It should be noticed that this ambitious goal stood in clear opposition to the common tendency in the Israeli army, until the 1973 War, to silence and censure expressions of mental distress among soldiers (Bilu and Witztum, 2000; Solomon, 1993). However, even the shift in terms of recognition and professional aid to trauma victims that occurred in the wake of the turmoil the country went through after the war (Solomon, 1993) was still a far cry from the broad scope NATAL experts had in mind. By launching the new project, the experts from NATAL stopped referring to trauma and PTSD as the pathology of a handful of individuals who had developed clinical symptoms, and started attributing it to the absolute majority. Encompassed in this group was every soldier who had participated, in one way or another, in the events of the Intifada. In light of this new expanded boundary, a much more positive and normative marker, "graduates of friction," replaced the clinical marker of "disorder."

Despite the ambitious start, the attempt to vitalize the project quickly proved to be especially challenging. The initial advertisements in the media and on the NGO website did not generate a critical mass of applications by discharged soldiers asking for NATAL's therapeutic services. As a result, alongside the first classic practice of (1) *treatment* in the clinic, three others were gradually employed as (2) *documentation* of combat soldiers' and POWs' personal narratives, (3) qualitative and quantitative *research* among discharged soldiers, and finally, (4) a proactive *search* of students who had served in the reserves during the Second Intifada. In what follows, I present these four practices – *treating, documenting, researching,* and *identifying* – and shed light on how dealing with trauma and PTSD among diverse groups of soldiers served not only as a means of coping with the moral questions that military service posed to soldiers themselves but also as an optional answer to questions posed to the entire Jewish-Israeli society.

Treating: From Moral Drama to Emotional Drama

Faithful to the primal meaning of trauma in the context of the Arab–Israeli conflict, the therapists sought to encourage discharged soldiers to accept clinical treatment in order to avoid a recurrence of what they usually called "the Yom Kippur generation." Those who had fought in the 1973 War (also known as the Yom Kippur War), out of shame or unawareness, did not receive mental therapy even when their fighting experience had left ghastly memories and had impaired their lives. When they did come, if they did, it was too late, from the therapists' point of view, to assist them effectively.

Two soldiers who did respond to NATAL's solicitation were Udi and Oren. The way NATAL's clinical staff interpreted both stories demonstrates the translation of moral drama into emotional drama and the debates and disagreements that had evolved from this process of translation. As an anthropologist, I was able to track ethnographically how this process played out through one of the important resources at the therapists' disposal: the "case presentation" during the team's clinical meetings. Often in therapeutic work, the team members convene biweekly meetings. According to a predetermined order, each team member presents a narrative of a patient, the "case," and asks his or her colleagues and superiors to give feedback. In all the case presentations conducted during the team meetings, what stood out was the therapists' attempts to translate the patients' stories of distress into the diagnostic category of trauma and its narrative structure. However, since the stories originated from a violent political conflict, certain components of the mental injury frequently challenged the process of translation and exposed how the politics of trauma were intermingling with the context of the clinic.

Udi: "He was defending himself and I put a bullet in his head"

In November 2005, Nimrod Dror, a clinical psychologist, presented the case of one of his new patients, Udi. Speaking at length, Dror delivered bits of information about Udi: single, parents divorced; father with a new family; mother unemployed, remarried but no children; has learning difficulties; unable to fall in love or live conjugally; previously lived in the United States, India, and Australia; smokes drugs and drinks alcohol. Dror then dwelled upon one particular incident during which Udi's army unit had engaged with another IDF unit. According to Dror, the two units had not practised together prior to going into action, which led to mistaken and deadly fire by Udi, as he told the therapist:

> "While clearing a route we were engaged, and because we hadn't practised together, we fired at the other unit and assaulted them." He leapt

over a low wall of stones; the major of the other unit was lying on the
ground; he'd been hit. "And when I saw him with the rifle, I shot several
rounds into his chest. He defended himself, threw his arms over his head,
and I put a bullet in his head." (13 November 2005, Field Notes)

This mistaken shooting of a comrade who was holding up his arms in
surrender and its lethal outcome, certainly fit the definition of "an exceptional triggering event" as it appears in the iconic classification of
PTSD. Later on, the therapist described this event as having wreaked
havoc in Udi's life and as having impaired his functioning. Dror said
that Udi continued to suffer from "recurrent images when he hears reports about skirmishes and can hardly sleep, worried about what the
future holds," and that he was angry and frustrated to the point of
"wanting to take a punching bag and slam into it." Dror presented the
traumatic event, and the marks it left on Udi's soul, as such that it justified going into therapy:

> During our first meeting I saw a slender young man, thinning hair, black
> rings under his eyes, projecting a deep and vast sadness ... He talks about
> wanting to get out of the situation ... Actually, he can't get himself up off the
> sofa ... When he was thinking of cancelling a meeting with me, I texted him
> a message: "You decide." He texted me back: "The last time I decided, I
> killed someone I wasn't supposed to kill." (13 November 2005, Field Notes)

The translation of Udi's story, from the sociopolitical context in which it
occurred into the diagnostic category of PTSD, is clear and convincing:
a distinctive and unusual triggering factor led to a series of mental
symptoms. The therapy also served its initial purpose of allowing the
patient to remember the traumatic material and observe the connection between it and early childhood experiences. However, the debate
among the team members showed that even when there is a high degree of accord between the patient's story and the disorder's clinical
nucleus, a negotiation rapidly develops. First to speak was Dr. Shai
Gur, the team's psychiatrist:

> DR. SHAI GUR (PSYCHIATRIST): It sounds like there's a problem in
> understanding the cause. He [the patient] strongly connects action with
> aggression, and also acts that way. Even the central traumatic event
> sounds as if there was something he did that's beyond [a problem of]
> practice.

TZIPI ROT (CLINICAL PSYCHOLOGIST): I suppose you could see if [the victim] was one of our soldiers. I don't know. I've never been in combat.

DR. GUR: [More than in other areas, the military activity in] Lebanon arouses feelings of helplessness, whether they [objectively] exist or not. It seems to me there are too many [functional] things [in Udi's life] that you have to treat before the [emotional and] dynamic parts.

DR. BARNEA (CHIEF PSYCHOLOGIST): He [the patient] is delivering a message that can paralyze: helplessness and being overactive ... He killed someone ... For me the difficult part was that he said that the other young man raised his arms, and he shot him in the head. And I also know where that difficulty inside me comes from.[1]

MICHAL LEIFER (SOCIAL WORKER): What do you do with a patient who has killed? What happens to us [as therapists] when we face someone in whom we discover aggression? It isn't simple facing patients. Sorrow and pain, that's simpler, but these places, they aren't simple.

LISA KIRON (DANCE THERAPIST): There is a very great difficulty, when inside the trauma there is a component of aggression and guilt, as opposed to trauma that happened to him. (13 November 2005, Field Notes)

The above exchange among the team members reveals how complicated it was to translate a military and moral drama, the mistaken killing of a comrade whose arms were raised in surrender, into a psychological drama. The team members perceived the triggering factor for PTSD, namely, the problematic nature of the killing, as containing a dimension of aggression that could not be dismissed as a lack of practice; for even in its absence, as one of the therapists said, "you could see if [the victim] was one of our soldiers." Therefore, even though Udi's mental state was a perfect match for the diagnostic category of PTSD, Udi did not fit the parameters of "pure victim" (Malkki, 1996), the person who should and ought to be helped. He was not someone who had had aggression directed at him, as the dance therapist argued, but rather he himself had been the aggressor by mistakenly opening fire and killing.

---

1 As he said several times in professional forums and in a personal interview I conducted with him (27 July 2005), Dr. Itamar Barnea had been a repatriated POW. During the 1973 War, he served as a pilot in the Israeli Air Force, was shot down and badly wounded, and spent eight months in Syrian captivity.

Barnea, NATAL's chief psychologist, hinted at Udi's problematic position as a victim of trauma, noting that he had shot a man in the head who had been surrendering. One of the therapists, Michal Leifer, further amplified the jarring discord between the position of "patient" and the expression of lethal aggression by asking: "What do you [as therapists] do with a patient who has killed?"

However, against this challenge to Udi's legitimate position as a patient, some of the team members posited the therapeutic imperative to avoid judgment, a quality which is identified as a central component of clinical practice. Sa'ar Uzieli, for example, the team leader, argued:

> He could have won renown for himself, because if it had been a terrorist he would have come out a hero. He acted impeccably. The situation is so chaotic, two forces engaging each other, pandemonium. In the heat of the moment, it's either him or me. It's a split second in which you have to make a decision. Precisely in a case where he was on the ball, something terrible happened. It doesn't matter what he does, even if it's appropriate, it's bad. That's the trauma. (13 November 2005, Field Notes)

In his remarks, the team leader sought to avoid judging Udi too harshly and, in that, to re-establish Udi's legitimate position as a victim of trauma and as a patient. For that purpose, Uzieli made use of a social argument, not a clinical argument (e.g., the emotional turmoil besetting Udi). The organizational "pandemonium" ensuing from the engagement of two units in a combat situation served as sufficient explanation for the mistaken fire and justified why Udi should not be tagged as an exceptional patient, "a patient who killed."

Oren: "The Ministry of Defense as an object of projection"

In January 2006, another of the team's therapists, Tal Rabinowitz, presented the case of Oren, who had been a combat soldier in the army and who had a particularly difficult relationship with his father. Rabinowitz spoke of what had led Oren to seek therapy:

> They entered a Palestinian village in two armored trucks and one of them [the trucks] started burning. A large crowd gathered ... He spotted five armed Palestinians, jumped out of the truck, got his footing, shot them in the legs. They fled and he received a mark of distinction. But questions arose in him as to whether he could have harmed them less. In [Operation]

Defensive Shield there was great tension and uncertainty. He noticed a man who looked dangerous to him. He shot at him, but didn't know if he hit him or not. The face of that young man keeps coming back to him. [At the start of his military service] he [mistakenly] squeezed off a bullet one time ... During the course, in the first drill, he almost ran over comrades who were waiting for them. (22 January 2006, Field Notes)

As can be seen, Oren's story was missing the unequivocal triggering factor so apparent in Udi's story. The therapist described a series of events in which Oren made use of a weapon. From her viewpoint, these incidents amounted to a critical mass that yielded a diagnosis of PTSD. Their negative mental effect on his life became apparent later. The therapist presented a series of symptoms from which Oren was suffering, going on to describe how the therapy was helping him process the traumatic experiences:

For half a year, he has had a girlfriend. The communication and intimacy are developing more and more, but he finds it hard to set limits. He does things that lead to arguments and are distancing ... He showed her pictures of sexual poses with his former girlfriend ... He has disturbing thoughts about harming himself, about injuries and blood. Thoughts also have begun to crop up about harming his girlfriend and his brother ... I pointed to the opposition between his weakness and the power he was given in the army ... I suggested to Oren that he is unable to separate the external reality of war, in which people shoot and harm others and are harmed themselves, from his own inner reality ... I suggested to him that [when he is shooting] a rubber bullet – his goal is to set a limit if people don't follow [his] instructions. (22 January 2006, Field Notes)

As in Udi's case, a process took place of translating the moral drama in which Oren had participated while serving in the army into an emotional one. From describing the actual harm to the Palestinians, the therapist shifted to describing the imaginary harm to his girlfriend, his brother, and himself. However, as opposed to Udi's case, the team members proceeded with this translation in a more relaxed manner. Unlike Udi, who had mistakenly shot a comrade, the excess aggression that Oren had exhibited towards Palestinians did not call into question his legitimate position as a "pure victim" of trauma and as a patient. Furthermore, the moral drama in which he had participated in the military context served as an explanatory metaphor for the emotional drama of his intimate relations with his girlfriend. As such, the therapist interpreted the shooting of rubber bullets as an attempt "to set a limit if people don't follow instructions," whether they be Palestinians or his girlfriend.

However, doubt crept into what seemed to be a complete translation into the diagnostic category of PTSD from an unexpected direction. Towards the end of the case presentation, Rabinowitz explained that at one of their most recent meetings, Oren had shared with her his intention of using his PTSD diagnosis to file a lawsuit against the Ministry of Defense. While she supported her diagnosis of his condition as post-traumatic, the therapist asked the question that was troubling her: "Is it right to help him with the forms for the [lawsuit] against the Ministry of Defense? To encourage or raise the questions of guilt vis-à-vis the [army] system?"

> SA'AR UZIELI (THE HEAD OF THE TEAM): It's not certain that he'll be recognized by the Ministry of Defense. He's liable to be disappointed … He is angriest at the place from which he received the least recognition: from his father. And if he isn't recognized by the father and won't be recognized by the Ministry of Defense – that'll be a problem. And the question is, will he be able to deal with [the double] rejection?
>
> UDIT ROM (CLINICAL PSYCHOLOGIST): What he's doing vis-à-vis the Ministry of Defense – non-recognition might take [him] to a very difficult place. The ability to ask for recognition, "Look at me," at whom is it actually directed? The Ministry of Defense is just an object of projection, and the Ministry of Defense is a problematic object of projection.
>
> SA'AR UZIELI: It's important to deal with him. He only wants to be seen, that room be made for him, that he be told that it's right. And it has to happen inside him. If you [the therapist] could deal with what's happening with him, then he'll understand that he doesn't need this [the Defense Ministry's] recognition. That should be [your] message [to him].
> (22 January 2006, Field Notes)

The team members thus sought to avoid translating the clinical diagnosis back into the social context. They did not interpret Oren's intention of claiming recognition as a legitimate attempt to translate the clinical diagnosis into an economic gain, but rather saw it as a "transference" of his desire to win recognition from his father. Oren's attainment of a higher level of self-awareness, which could result from therapy, might make the need for that recognition unnecessary.

Documenting: Steven Spielberg in the IDF Uniform

My parents came from Czechoslovakia. They went through the Holocaust. In our family, no one likes to mention the Holocaust. In our house, we were always thinking about the future, not thinking about the past. No one ever wants to remember what was. What *will be* is more interesting.

– David Levin, documentation project, NATAL, 2010

These are the opening remarks in the testimony given by David – a second-generation Holocaust survivor, a combat soldier in the 1973 War, and a repatriated POW – to a NATAL clinical psychologist. David was one of several dozen combat soldiers who answered NATAL's invitation to testify about their military service experiences. Without conscious intention, David cross-referenced two situations: the silenced testimony by his parents as Holocaust survivors in front of their children, and his own testimony as a combat soldier in the Israeli army in front of the psychologist.

David's testimony, alongside those of another few dozen combat soldiers, provided the foundation for a project whose declared purpose was to "duplicate" the American documentation project on Holocaust survivors, funded by Steven Spielberg.

The project was the first creative attempt to have Israeli soldiers and repatriated POWs from different generations recognize that their mental injuries were the result of their military service. This occurred within the framework of the broader professional effort to garner public recognition of security-based trauma in Israel. This endeavour, as can be seen, clearly exceeded the bounds of classic therapy. NATAL formulated the proposal for soldiers and repatriated POWs as an invitation to take part in a "documentation" project, not as an invitation to receive mental aid; to tell their personal story to a psychologist in front of a camera. NATAL senior staff set two primary goals for this documentation effort. The first goal was to have the participants undergo some kind of personal process. Even though it did not occur in "therapy," hopefully, the recollection of harsh experiences from military service or captivity in a structured narrative setting in response to a psychologist's questions would help the individual process the traumatic content. The second goal was social. "This is a psycho-historic project," a NATAL senior expert clarified at a steering committee meeting (11 April 2011, Field Notes). The steering committee hoped the testimonies of the participants would amount to a collective mosaic from a personal perspective about events in Israel's history.

Sociocultural analysis of ten of the testimonies opened a peep-hole into the tension that had arisen between the clinical concerns of NATAL's testimony project and the social circumstances surrounding it. A stubborn struggle ensued between the testimonies of the partici-pants and the context in which they were delivered – the treatment room. Most of the participants, like David, did not use trauma (or PTSD) as an organizing interpretative scheme for their stories. In the face of the psychologist's questions, they posed resistance through the use of various social codes identified with masculine identity in Israel (see Lieblich, 1978; Lomsky-Feder, 2004). David's parents, by their si-lence, had refused to give expression to the mental trauma they had experienced during the Holocaust. Accordingly, he chose to open his testimony by trying to mark it as unnecessary: the future is the im-portant, the interesting time. The past, the time on which the act of testimony rests, is idle time; it is the time that has been and, therefore, is less important and less interesting. Similarly, the testimonies of the other participants did not provide a bridge to their inner psychic world. Rather, it turned out to be an opportunity to flaunt various codes of masculinity, such as the values of rationality and dignity.

Danny, for example, who had fought in the 1973 War, described one of the most dramatic moments for him as follows:

> The moment I saw there was no Israeli flag, and I saw the Egyptian flag – I said that's it. It's the conclusion of a chapter. At this moment we're losing this war. And then the chapter of fear of death ended as well. Your head becomes bright and clear, and you start thinking with incredible cool: the knowledge that you're going to die is already sitting there [in your mind].

Danny delivered a testimony expressing his personal experience by focusing on a group element – nationalism. Israel's most distinctive symbol, the national flag, was wrapped up with feelings and thoughts of "self": replacing the Israeli flag with the Egyptian flag marked the conclusion of the chapter of "fear of death," and the start of the chap-ter of "thinking with incredible cool." However, precisely the most distinctive raw materials that comprise PTSD, terrible fright joined with the absolute helplessness of a lonely soldier facing enemy forces, demonstrated Danny's value of rationality in his testimony: "thinking with incredible cool," with regard to "the knowledge that you're going to die."

Eyal, to take another example, fought in the Second Lebanon War. Like Danny, he sought to describe his grave fear of death by rationally detaching himself from his family, rather than by expressing feelings identified with trauma. He explained a decision he reached when he was returning to his military unit after a weekend at home with his wife and children:

> I simply disconnect from them ... I've simply said goodbye to the family ... I'm with my soldiers. I'm full of energy, functioning. I completely disconnected from the family emotionally. I hardly ever telephoned [them] ... I can't be in a place where I have to function at my best and where I could die, and on the other hand – the family. It doesn't go together.

The effectiveness of using social codes (like rationality) as an alternative way of interpreting harsh wartime experiences, rather than using the term "trauma," was further refined in regard to the experience of captivity. In line with Lomsky-Feder's (2004) findings on the soldiers of the 1973 War, the repatriated POWs who participated in NATAL's documentation project made sure to normalize their experiences and integrate them into the routine of their lives. For example, Avi, who had been in Egyptian captivity, stated: "In the course of my life, I've had an experience of captivity, an experience of war, an experience of heroism." Nadav, another repatriated POW, emphasized his attempt to achieve swift self-control while falling into captivity and afterwards. To the psychologist's question about the mental hardships that captivity entails, he quickly replied: "You'll hear sadder stories than mine ... I don't let things get to me. Maybe it's not good, but that's how I am." When asked to refer to the consequences of captivity for his subsequent life, Nadav chose to underscore simple positive ones: his longing to be free; to drive into the city from the kibbutz where he lives when he feels like it; to take a nap on Saturday afternoon even if there are guests.

Danny, the combat soldier who described how he replaced "the fear of death" with "thoughts of incredible cool," was also a POW. He was the only one on his military base who had survived when Egyptian forces captured him. NATAL's project directors often described Danny's testimony as especially revealing. As opposed to other POWs, Danny gave more details about the experience of captivity and the physical violence to which his Egyptian interrogators subjected him. However, this description exposed a different view of captivity from the traumatic one. For example, Danny described an especially long and harsh episode of violence as follows:

I couldn't feel my body at all, uncontrollable trembling. I was plastered to the floor. My legs gave out. And I knew – this is where the red line passes. That's it; [you should] know that this is what you're capable of suffering. Up to here.

Even from the distance of time, Danny's attitude towards the extreme violence he had experienced rested on a very rapid translation of his complete helplessness in captivity into a rational course of self-examination. Danny described his body as being "plastered to the floor," of experiencing "uncontrollable trembling" and his legs giving out. However, from his point of view, this suffering did not provide a basis for the description of mental trauma but led to a process of drawing conclusions. Danny used his suffering to learn about his own powers of endurance and to try to achieve a certain, albeit small, measure of control; to retain a certain, albeit small, measure of human dignity. Other repatriated POWs also described their attempts to quickly establish anchors of control and a measure of certainty in a situation that was filled with uncertainty and lack of control. Instead of describing what went on in the interrogation rooms, some of them talked about the routine of meals, the first shower in captivity, or various ingenious ways to maintain personal hygiene. Others recalled a prison guard who had been more sensitive and who allowed the prisoners to recite the *Shema* (daily prayer), or the acts of a solicitous cellmate.

In delivering their testimonies, the combat soldiers and repatriated POWs did not help accomplish the first goal associated with the documentation. "Processing of mental trauma" was clearly missing from the testimonies they delivered. It was still too early to tell whether the second goal had been met, the "psycho-historic" documentation. However, it seemed that more than providing personal narratives of trauma, the subjects of the "Israeli Spielberg project" reaffirmed the old perception of masculinity in Israel, the one based on physical and mental strength.

Researching: Focus Groups versus Telephone Survey

In their continuing attempt to alter public opinion about trauma among IDF soldiers, NATAL therapists engaged in another practice: research. The rationale for the research rested on the post-Vietnam American context, and even more on the contemporary American wars in Iraq and Afghanistan. While the American public had become aware of the fact that its soldiers were involved in brutal behaviour in Vietnam, a clinical assumption was being established that the aggressors, and not only the victims, might suffer from mental trauma. This assumption developed to the point of yielding a specific category: "self-traumatized perpetrator," an individual who is both the aggressor and the victim of PTSD at the same time (see Young, 2002).

In light of this definition, NATAL experts sought to conduct a qualitative study among IDF soldiers in order to examine whether their engagement with the civilian Palestinian population during the First and Second Intifadas had indeed seared traumatic memories in their minds, different from those of soldiers who had fought against an army during the Wars of 1973 and 1982. The study was based on focus groups, by means of which they wanted "to learn in greater depth what the nature of the hardships [of discharged soldiers] is, and then we'll learn how to bring them [to the clinic]," as the head of NATAL's steering committee put it (28 September 2005, Field Notes).

In December 2005, two groups of discharged soldiers, one aged twenty-one to twenty-nine and another aged twenty-five to thirty-five, gathered at a research institute in central Israel. Earlier, an initial screening process took place to ensure the participants would define themselves as having undergone devastating or painful experiences during their military service. All NATAL senior experts and officials came to observe the focus groups, and I joined them. We sat in a small room, observing, through a one-way mirror, the questions being asked by the moderator and the answers being given by the participants, who were aware they were being watched:[2]

> MODERATOR: When you think about regular military service or the reserves, what pops into your head?
> ANSWERS: Green/Guard duty shifts/Being stuck/Being fed up/Friends/ Lots of sand/Adventure/Tension.
> MODERATOR: When you think about the encounter with the Palestinian population, what comes to mind?
> ANSWERS: Arrests/Roadblocks/Anger/Stones/Difficult mental situations/Taking their anger out on us/Shame at what we've come to.

---

2 To facilitate the dialogue of these exchanges, different short answers have been compiled into a single paragraph and separated by slashes. More elaborate answers are presented separately.

MODERATOR: Let's focus on the negative experiences. Tell me a little.

ANSWERS: Confrontations/Stones being thrown/Seeing soldiers get hurt. That's the hardest part.

MODERATOR: From what aspect?

1ST PARTICIPANT: Seeing a friend that you've spent a considerable amount of time with, to see that he's hurting and struggling. It makes me feel bad, makes me hate the people who threw stones. Rage, anger.

2ND PARTICIPANT: At the roadblocks you see people who are very scared, and you're scared too. You don't know how to behave, it's all based on the mood, helplessness. You would prefer not to be a part of it, like before the army. I don't really share [these stories]. You've carved out a way of looking at things for yourself. You don't share, and nobody's a saint either.

3RD PARTICIPANT: I've shared with friends who've experienced it, an arrest inside a Palestinian village. As soon as you go in, a search for weapons is conducted, and after we've rounded up the family, then small children, or somebody just like you, only from the other side, and someone aims a rifle at them, a mother and baby and a grandmother. It's only in the army that you can see such things. And you tell your friends. It's hard to open up unless it's someone who was there.

4TH PARTICIPANT: I don't think that sharing can offer any help, unless it concerns an especially traumatic experience. These are routine matters. People who are with me are familiar with it like me. Other people can't help you. I've chosen it. It can't console or help.

MODERATOR: You say that someone who wasn't there is less able to understand. Did you feel that the experience of friction with the Palestinian population was leaching into your day-to-day lives even after you left the field?

1ST PARTICIPANT: With me, yes, because I saw things that they [the Palestinians] were really miserable. Manning the frontline in Hebron, there were contacts between the Haredim [ultra-Orthodox Jews] and wearers of knitted yarmulkes [National Orthodox], who would stir up trouble themselves. Afterwards, when you see the pictures on television, you know that the ones stirring up trouble are the Haredim themselves. The Palestinians are careworn people, who go through five to six roadblocks every day.

MODERATOR: Just a moment, gentlemen, you're telling me about the Palestinian population and that's fine, but I'd like to hear about yourselves.

ANSWERS: I have a friend who has nightmares in his head./I have a friend who keeps quitting his job, constantly has outbursts and yells./

In civilian life, you're in a different framework, and that causes
flashbacks, helplessness. When you go in you see that they aren't
innocent and they aren't miserable. (4 December 2005, Field Notes)

The above exchange illustrates how the moderator tried to promote a
specific interpretation of the participants' military service. What stood
out against the multidimensionality exhibited by their answers regarding military service ("Green," "Being fed up," "Friends," "Adventure,"
or "Tension") was the moderator's focus on a single aspect: the negative experience of their encounter with the Palestinians. Indeed, this
focus did reveal a mental vulnerability among the soldiers. They described experiences of fear, pain, anger, frustration, and guilt. Some of
them affirmed that the source of the vulnerability was twofold: alongside the threat that they felt to themselves, they described the difficulty
of behaving in a way that caused suffering to civilians, including groups
identified as particularly vulnerable such as babies and the aged.

From this point on, however, there was a split between the moderator's mode of understanding the meaning of the mental difficulties
and the participants' mode of understanding it. Whereas most of them
chose to position the Palestinian suffering at the centre, the moderator
wanted them to focus on their own suffering. Yet even those who com-
plied with this request, associated their mental vulnerability with "routine," "choice," or "a part of you," and felt no urgent need to share it
with others. The moderator sought to ascertain their willingness to define their hardships as mental distress that required professional help:

MODERATOR: I'll state names of organizations in Israel that provide aid
   to soldiers. Please share with me your associations with each of them.
   The Ministry of Defense.
ANSWERS: Disability/Work/Release/Army/[Financial] Conditions/
   Government.
MODERATOR: To what extent does the Ministry of Defense help one cope?
1ST PARTICIPANT: Only if you come out with a very traumatic disability.
MODERATOR: What needs does it answer?
2ND PARTICIPANT: Financial. It points to the right places.
MODERATOR: And NATAL?
3RD PARTICIPANT: It's more to help families; with loss, with terror
   attacks, with traumatic situations.
4TH PARTICIPANT: One of the things that's disturbing when there's a
   mental problem is that you don't want to feel mentally ill. You don't

want to see mothers and children, because then you aren't miserable enough. You're relatively okay. I would prefer to be with soldiers and not with other populations. (4 December 2005, Field Notes)

The moderator's ongoing effort to impose a specific pattern of interpretation on the military service of the participants – as a cause of mental distress that requires professional assistance – ran aground. Most of the participants preferred to keep their harsh experiences to themselves and were in no hurry to identify themselves as "in need" of mental aid. It emerged that the young discharged soldiers, like the older combat soldiers and repatriated POWs, embodied the common Israeli concept of masculinity (see Lomsky-Feder, 2004): the man who serves in the army is physically and mentally strong. From their viewpoint, whoever needs mental aid must be suffering from "a very traumatic disability," which they identified with "mothers and children," two groups that do not actively participate in the battlefield. They identified themselves, indirectly, as the polar opposite of these two groups, and expressed a reluctance to identify themselves as "mentally ill."

In the absence of unequivocal findings from the focus groups, NATAL experts decided to conduct a telephone survey among a representative sample of several hundred discharged soldiers. The purpose of the survey was to assess more accurately how many soldiers, who had served in the Occupied Territories, had developed symptoms associated with trauma. The opening part of the telephone questionnaire was devoted to identifying the source of the soldier's suffering. Among NATAL senior staff members there was agreement regarding certain questions, such as the following: "Were you wounded while you were serving?" "Were you the victim of physical or verbal violence?" "Did you witness physical or verbal violence?" "Did you witness anything that seemed like humiliation to you?" "While serving did you ever risk death in the wake of a confrontation?"

However, there was no agreement regarding other questions, such as "Who made you a victim of physical or verbal violence?" and "Towards whom was the physical or verbal violence you witnessed directed?" In the first version of the questionnaire, the suggested phrasing was "by/towards Palestinian civilians." Professor Mark Gelkopf, the head researcher, explained: "There's a difference between a civilian and a combat soldier … Armed men have always been targeted for harm. What's interesting here [with the Intifada] is that it's vis-à-vis civilians" (Steering Committee, 4 January 2006, Field Notes).

This clinical-political argument quickly sparked an intense debate, and the process of drawing up the questionnaire became challenging. The assumption that Israeli soldiers might have PTSD originating from aggression on their part, rather than being victims of aggression, was enough to pose a real threat to the perception of the Israeli soldier as one who maintains humane ethical standards (see Solomon, 1993). The head of the clinical team, for example, argued with the researcher who thought the questionnaire should be focused on questions concerning harm to Palestinian civilians by asking, "What is a civilian? Isn't an Israeli soldier a civilian?" The researcher answered him, "No, according to the Geneva Convention, he is not a civilian!" Others expressed the concern that it might put the Israeli army and its soldiers in a negative light. "It's important it doesn't turn out that we're being unnecessarily violent towards civilians," said Barnea, NATAL's chief psychologist. "[The questionnaire should demonstrate] that we're also dealing with armed men."

Eventually, the questionnaire did refer to "Palestinian civilians," without specifying whether they were armed or not. Two hundred and forty soldiers responded to it: 170 soldiers who had come into contact with Palestinian civilians, and seventy who hadn't and who therefore served as a control group. A month later, at a meeting of the steering committee in February 2006, the researcher presented the main conclusion:

> There is a symptomatic profile. It's not some hibernating beast ... They have got to be provided information. We shouldn't be saying, "Come to be treated," "come to be treated," "come to be treated," but getting to them in another way. Giving [them] something more experiential. (15 February 2006, Field Notes)

The data collection process did not yield clear-cut conclusions. From the descriptions of the soldiers in the focus groups and from the findings of the telephone survey, a picture emerged that largely fit the subdiagnostic category of the "self-traumatized perpetrator." At the same time, the soldiers repeatedly manifested a tendency not to identify themselves as suffering from emotional hardship, and certainly not as the bearers of a mental disorder. From this stemmed their self-declared inclination to avoid seeking professional aid. This duality required the therapists to exercise high measures of caution in addressing the soldiers, while trying to figure out how to apply their psychological principles to this target audience. Therefore, they were looking for more neutral and non-psychological terms such as "experience" rather than persuading the soldiers to "be treated."

Identifying: "It's sacred work: Name by name, soldier by soldier"

The most creative practice NATAL therapists employed to expand the relevancy of trauma and PTSD to the IDF's soldiers, and by doing so to alter public recognition of it, was the proactive effort to identify discharged soldiers out of a concern that they might be suffering from post-traumatic symptoms. This ensued through an unusual collaboration between NATAL and the clinical department at one of Israel's large universities in the wake of the Second Lebanon War. The dean of students at the university provided the therapists at NATAL's hotline open access to 470 names and telephone numbers of students who reported having served in the reserves during the war. As opposed to treating, documenting, and researching, here NATAL commenced to identify students with no preliminary indication that any of them were suffering from traumatic symptoms.

The uniqueness of this practice emerged from a document distributed among NATAL hotline therapists, which read: "In the conversations that we shall initiate with the students, we'll be 'landing' on them without their being prepared for it ... *Furthermore – when it is not at all certain that they think they have any problem that requires and justifies such a conversation*" (italics in the original, NATAL Internal Document, 14 May 2007). In other words, just having participated in the war qualified them for participation in a "pre-clinical" group and, therefore, they should be contacted.

From the start, the therapists recognized that this exceptional step required a high level of caution. They needed to formulate and conduct the conversations with the students thoughtfully, as the document went on to explain:

> The conversation should begin with the question whether he has time to talk with us briefly. At this stage, and in light of the fact that we've contacted them without prior warning, we'll present our justification for having the conversation, and that is we understand that they served in the military reserves the past summer, and that we assume it wasn't an easy

time for them … We'd like to know how they're doing … If the students dismiss us with a reply of "Okay" or find it hard to answer, you can specify: Have they been able to return to concentrating on their schoolwork? How are they sleeping at night? … Are they able to study for their exams? Do they have outbursts of rage? … You should say that in our [professional] experience people who have undergone severe incidents of fighting or real threats to their lives may develop various symptoms that they should be aware of, and specify them. (NATAL Internal Document, 14 May 2007)

As can be seen, the guidelines regarding the calls clearly show how the diagnostic category of PTSD was "foisted" on the students top-down. It was clear to the therapists that it was very likely their calls would encounter resistance, so they developed various tactics in advance to overcome that. They used the most mundane phrasing to introduce the purpose of the call and to lay the ground for having the conversation at all. In response to the anticipated "Okay," they instructed hotline therapists to convey a gentle but clear warning about "various symptoms" by virtue of their professional experience. Hanna, a senior hotline therapist and one of the project leaders, described it as "sacred work: name by name, soldier by soldier" (interview, 20 August 2007).

Below I present two telephone calls conducted by a NATAL hotline therapist, one with Omer and one with Boris.[3] Both conversations occurred on the anniversary of the outbreak of the Second Lebanon War.

Conversation with Omer

THERAPIST: Hello there … Being a year since the war, we are calling students who were in the war in order to hear how the year has gone by. What was the situation then? What's happening now? If you're willing to share a little.

---

3 As part of the ongoing monitoring of the project, I was permitted to listen in on the conversations between the therapist and the two students on a telephone extension. Similar to every other research action in the project, the soldiers' personal details, including name, age, place of residence, field of study, and service unit, have been deleted or disguised.

OMER: The truth is we happened to have a day of reserve duty after the war with a psychologist [from the army] and she was rather bored. No one in our unit was hurt, although we fought and have even now received a battalion citation. We don't have experiences of terrible fear or such things, so I don't have too much to tell. We simply worked by the book, so we prevented loss of life.

THERAPIST: It's good they talked with you ... You say that you "worked by the book." I can hear the fraternity.

OMER: When you are in such places, then there's no choice but to be together. There's no desire to make it harder than it is. There was a very good [social] atmosphere. It's important that you trust in your friends as in yourself, because if not then we'll all be in trouble. Alone, we can't fight. There's no Rambo in the IDF.

THERAPIST: I'm glad it was a good experience.

OMER: Yes, you could call it a good experience, certainly.

THERAPIST: We want to raise awareness of the possibility of traumatic injury, because that's part of being able to go out to battle in better form.

OMER: Yes, I've already done reserve duty after the war and now I'm going again.

THERAPIST: And there haven't been any signs of sleeping problems, problems with concentration?

OMER: No, truthfully no.

THERAPIST: Omer, thank you very much, and be well. (20 August 2007, Field Notes)

Omer explicitly rejected the therapist's attempt to situate his experiences from the war within the sphere of trauma. While the therapist addressed him by using the singular voice ("you"), Omer chose to speak in the plural ("us"). He referred to fighting as a group experience that was performed based on trust, training, and comradeship. He pointed out that even the psychologist sent by the army to talk with them after the war "was rather bored," perhaps like the one now talking to him on the telephone. Omer stuck to the group interpretation of his participation in the war, even when the therapist suggested harnessing the awareness of mental trauma for more efficient functioning during combat.

The second student whom the therapist contacted that day was Boris. As will emerge from the conversation, not only did Boris serve in the reserves during the war but he was also a resident living in the north, so he had experienced rocket fire firsthand.

Conversation with Boris

THERAPIST: Hello there ... Being a year since the war, we are calling
students who were in the war, in order to hear how the year has gone by.

BORIS: What exactly are you interested in? What, are you filling in a
questionnaire?

THERAPIST: No, no, no. It's a service for students, to see if there's a need
for help.

BORIS: What? Conversation? A psychologist?

THERAPIST: Yes, there is such a service if there's a need. We want to
present the possibility.

BORIS: The truth is I've taken a break from my studies. After the war,
I had a financial problem, and only afterwards did they notify me that
I'd received a grant ... Everything's okay, nothing special. I can't say that
I've lost my concentration or anything like that. I was in the reserves for
a month, and except for financial hardships, there was nothing much.

THERAPIST: Because it isn't simple.

BORIS: No, it isn't. The entire country is one big army, and you've got
to help.

THERAPIST: Is your family in the northern region as well?

BORIS: Yes, I was in Haifa, and the building in which my future wife lived
took a direct hit ... I didn't want to leave, but a rocket simply hit her
building, and from there I was already called up to the reserves.

THERAPIST: What's important to us is to raise awareness. This is a
different war. The hinterland took part in it. We were all under the same
umbrella. It's also a collective trauma.

BORIS: I'm not sure about "everyone." There were Arabs at the university
who were happy the rockets were falling. But the majority, yes.

THERAPIST: Have you gone back to your routine? Haven't felt any
difficulty?

BORIS: No, no, not at all, thank God it's all over. Many people I know were
hurt, because they were around where the rockets struck ...

THERAPIST: Thank you. Goodbye. (20 August 2007, Field Notes)

Despite his twofold vulnerability (reserve service during the war and a
rocket strike on his girlfriend's building), Boris, like Omer, dismissed
symptoms of PTSD. Right from the start, he showed suspicion regarding the therapist's call, trying to ascertain whether the conversation
might serve the needs of the caller more than his own. Like Omer, Boris
also made use of the plural voice ("The entire country is one big army"),

but when the therapist tried to describe the war as "a collective trauma," he referred to Israel's unique demographic structure, claiming, "There were Arabs at the university who were happy the rockets were falling." As opposed to Omer, Boris did admit to significant hardship after the war, albeit financial and not mental.

Conclusion

The return of the therapists from their more liberated social location as members of an NGO to the place where the awareness of mental trauma in Israel had started to develop, the IDF, exposed the politics and pragmatics that were swirling around the clinical nucleus of the disorder. As illustrated, the therapists employed four different practices in reference to the military experiences of combat soldiers over the generations: treating, documenting, researching, and identifying. By doing so, high degrees of creativity, improvisation, and flexibility were expressed which made it possible to adapt trauma into a more contemporary concept to deal with the weighty moral questions that military service poses to Israeli society. Thus, the experts have constantly extended their scope of activity. They expanded from treating individuals who served in the IDF and were diagnosed with post-traumatic symptoms (treating), to therapeutic activities with large groups of soldiers (documenting and researching), to professional screening of soldiers after the Second Lebanon War (identifying). From the first practice to the fourth, the experts' pattern of activity contained a tension between two poles: screening traumatic symptoms to find specific individuals suffering from a disorder, and treating them *versus* casting a general psychological gaze on an entire group of Israeli soldiers and marking them as carrying traumatic memories without any diagnostic process.

The classic practice of treatment revealed how a process of translation was occurring when the moral drama became an emotional one, by creating a fit between the combat soldier's military story and the diagnostic category of trauma. However, this process became blurry in two different situations. The first occurred in Udi's situation when the triggering factor for the trauma threatened the patient's legitimate position as a "pure victim" (Malkki, 1996). The second was Oren's situation, when the combat soldier sought to engage in an additional process beyond the therapy, but in the opposite direction: from the emotional drama based on his PTSD diagnosis, back to the moral drama, via his choice to file a lawsuit against the Ministry of Defense. In both cases, the therapists ultimately sought to adhere to their clinical principles, while avoiding – easily or hardly at all – any moral judgment.

The three other practices – documentation, research, and identification – were a creative attempt to slowly and cautiously draw away from dealing directly with traumatic symptoms inside the clinic for the sake of moving towards a much broader goal: the essence of being a Jewish man in Israel. This gradual process should be understood in light of the change that the local mental health establishment underwent regarding the mental suffering of combat soldiers. Since the 1973 War, therapists both in and out of the IDF criticized the silencing and censoring that had characterized their predecessors' attitude towards the mental suffering of soldiers during Israel's first decades. As opposed to the tendency to dismiss their behaviour as an expression of personal weakness, moral fault, or defeatism, the new generation of Israeli therapists pointed to the grave mental suffering among many of the soldiers (Bilu and Witztum, 2000; Solomon, 1993). In that sense, the professional engagement of NATAL with the mental condition of trauma among the IDF's soldiers was consistent with a general movement in Israel.

However, from their new position in civil society, the therapists from NATAL took a significant turn: they sought to see military service itself as a period of time and as a series of experiences that carry within them traumatic memories, without necessarily having a connection to any version of diagnostic process. This interpretation was not to be underestimated, neither in the context of the IDF nor the American military. Despite some major differences between these military organizations, efforts to recognize and help American veterans suffering from traumatic symptoms also conflicted with core values such as toughness and self-control. When a veteran was diagnosed with PTSD, it was usually accompanied by a social stigma (Finley, 2015; Kirmayer, 2015).

Against this background, it should be noticed how creative NATAL's engagement with the mental condition of trauma among soldiers was. The combination of various therapeutic practices extended trauma management from a strict psychiatric disorder into a more flexible social category aimed not at the pathological minority but at the normative majority. As such, the therapists provided an explanatory model for understanding moral, social, and emotional difficulties with which the soldiers directly, and all of Israeli society indirectly, were contending. The trauma that military service entailed was interpreted not merely as a narrow psychiatric diagnosis but was redefined through practices such as documenting and identifying. Accordingly, it has been turned into a social experience that carries symbolic weight in shaping the identity of discharged soldiers as adults, as students coping with exams, as potential spouses, and as fathers.

Furthermore, the addition of documentation, research, and identification to the classic practice of treatment has made the contact between the therapists and various groups of discharged soldiers much more frequent and less bound by strict criteria. The documentation of repatriated POWs stories, research among focus groups, and telephone calls to students who served during the Second Lebanon War were not subject to the clear rules that usually characterize the therapeutic relationship. Instead, these events took place in more fluid situations in terms of the discursive rules. For precisely that reason, these situations excelled in turning the mental cost that military service exacts into a locus around which a vivid and vibrant debate ensued.

This negotiation yielded a conflict in perspectives within each of the practices. First, with documenting, the traumatic framing of combat and captivity experiences clashed with a social code embedded with "masculine" traits of rationality and human dignity. Second, with researching, the therapeutic framing of the "self-traumatized perpetrator" from military interactions with the Palestinian population contrasted with more collective concepts of routine and fortitude. Third, with proactive identifying, the therapeutic framing of the reserve service experience during the Second Lebanon War through the definition of trauma collided with an interpretation that emphasized the group nature of war. Throughout these conflicts, the therapists made use of the clinical nucleus of trauma and its byproducts to conduct a freer investigation into the social and moral meaning of young men's participation in a violent political conflict and its mental consequences. Perhaps to their surprise, they encountered the all too familiar attributes of masculine identity as shaped by the army in Israeli society (Bilu and Witztum, 2000; Lieblich, 1978; Lomsky-Feder, 2004), as well as a similar dynamic in the U.S. (Finley, 2015; Kirmayer, 2015).

In the next chapter, I shall track another encounter between therapists and patients, but this time it is one step beyond the clinical nucleus of the trauma: the clinical concept of secondary trauma as experienced by the wives of men diagnosed with PTSD.

Chapter Five

Man, Woman, and Disorder:
Trauma in the Intimate Sphere of the Family

I am trying to see how I can extricate myself from this marriage, how to say goodbye ... I am no longer willing to understand, to support, and to be there for him ... I've never been in such a nightmare in my whole life. I take sleeping pills because he infuriates me. He makes me crazy. "Give me a kiss." "Give me a hug," [he says] ... For half a year already, I haven't slept next to him ... I can't be with him anymore, not out of pity and not by force.

> – Dalit, participant of a support group for women married
> to men diagnosed with PTSD, 14 October 2007

These remarks by Dalit, a participant of a support group for Jewish-Israeli women married to men diagnosed with security-based PTSD, shed light on the dramatic movement of the disorder from the primary victim, the man, to the one closest to him, his spouse. Her sleepless nights that push her to the point of using drugs, her unwillingness to share a bed with him, and ultimately her desire to leave him are all strong and painful evidence of how PTSD and its symptoms percolate from the man to his spouse, turning her into a new object of therapeutic intervention.

The recognition of the need to provide mental assistance to women married to men diagnosed with PTSD is not unique to Israel. Contemporary clinical research on trauma indicates that the consequences of life-threatening events are not limited to the direct victim but often affect his "significant others" who may eventually be diagnosed with secondary trauma. First in the context of the Vietnam War (Jordan et al., 1992), and later in the context of the wars in Iraq and Afghanistan (Milliken et al., 2007; Sayers et al., 2009), therapists have dealt with both male veterans and their female partners, emphasizing the importance of supporting the women during the men's rehabilitation. At the same time, they reported that the wives often experienced some form of severe distress that led to traumatic symptoms that were similar to those of their husbands. Based on those findings, therapists strongly recommended that "any assistance offered to men with PTSD must take into account supporting and empowering the wives and children" (Dekel et al., 2005: 34).

However, a support group for Jewish-Israeli women married to men diagnosed as suffering from PTSD provides an opportunity to examine the tense relations between primary and secondary trauma from a somewhat different angle. The far-reaching stigmatic effects of psychological collapse during military service influenced not only the construction of masculinity in Israel (Bilu and Witztum, 2000; Lieblich, 1978; Lomsky-Feder, 2004) but also the gender division of labour. While men were expected to participate as fearless soldiers in the army, the women were expected to fulfil their biological function of giving birth and raising children (Herzog, 1999; Moore, 2012; Sachs, Sa'ar, and Aharoni, 2007).

This chapter, therefore, examines the new dimension of politics that has evolved around trauma and PTSD in Israel: how clinical questions regarding post-traumatic symptoms and the risk of their transmission from husband to wife intersected with sociopolitical questions of gender power relations and intimacy within the family. In particular, I shed light on how the group's therapists have created a connection between using clinical labels and adhering to dominant gender expectations. Facing this explicit and implicit message, the participants actively used both clinical labels – PTSD and secondary trauma – to redefine their position vis-à-vis their spouses.

New Definitions, Old Love

Twelve Jewish women aged thirty-five to fifty-five years responded to NATAL's invitation to join a support group for wives whose husbands had been diagnosed with security-based PTSD. The initial purpose of the gathering was to learn how to cope with their husbands' symptoms so that they could not only better support them but also avoid developing secondary trauma symptoms themselves. Contrary to the official diagnosis of PTSD from the Ministry of Defense in the course of military service and from the National Insurance Institute in the event of a terrorist attack, the twelve women attended a preliminary clinical interview during which their needs and ability to benefit from such a therapeutic intervention were verified. There was no fee for participation, enabling the women, most of them from low-middle socio-economic backgrounds, to attend the meetings over an extended period. Two therapists led the group sessions: Dina, a clinical psychologist who had worked for years with families in the Israeli army, and Lin, an art therapist who was a senior lecturer at an Israeli college. Most sessions opened with each participant telling the group "where she's coming from today," which in many cases determined the rest of the session. In other sessions, one of the therapists presented a topic, often tied to family relationships, such as "childhood," "commitment," or "safe place," and asked the women to give it visual expression (through painting, sculpture, etc.), and to share their interpretations with the other women.

My entry into the group's sessions as an anthropologist was initiated by NATAL's senior staff. It was quite surprising in light of the original agreement that I would not conduct research activity in any clinical setting. However, two years of fieldwork prior to the gathering of the group led to the thought that qualitative research might provide another important viewpoint on the participants' experience. My acceptance by the participants was very quick. "Write it down, write it down," they would say to me. "It's important!" Indeed, throughout the two years of group sessions, I took detailed notes about the dynamic that took place between the participants and therapists. Furthermore, as a part of my agreement with the therapists, my notes from each session were typed and delivered to both the participants and therapists at the beginning of the following session.

In line with contemporary clinical literature (see Dekel et al., 2005; Jordan et al., 1992; Milliken et al., 2007; Sayers et al., 2009; Solomon, Dekel, and Zerach, 2008), the rationale that guided the group sessions was to teach the participants how to develop skills such as emotional exposure and emphatic communication, together with assertiveness, to help them cope with the changing circumstances of their marital relations. However, it quickly turned out that what was expected to be a neutral therapeutic process became highly enmeshed in gender power relations. Once the women became familiar with the clinical labels, they differed in how they interpreted the labels vis-à-vis their spouses. I demonstrate this diversity through the stories of Iris, Ayala, Michal, Hanna, and Dalit.

*Sleeping with a Disorder: "He used to be like a dog
in heat and now suddenly – nothing!"*

Yariv was a thirty-seven-year-old Israeli man who served in one of the
Israeli elite army units during the late 1980s. In line with the militaristic
orientation of Israel since its establishment in 1948 (Kimmerling, 1993),
stories of the unit's heroic operations are well known in local public
discourse. However, one afternoon, Iris, his thirty-five-year-old wife,
revealed another dimension of her husband's military service:

> [Yariv] suffered from dramatic collapses until he was completely apathet-
> ic. I didn't accept his behaviour. I didn't understand, until I read [about
> PTSD] on the internet … I saw my own life, one symptom after another.
> (9 March 2008, Field Notes)

As can be seen, Iris's understanding of Yariv's mental condition increased because she became familiar with the diagnostic category of
PTSD. The symptoms of the disorder, described on a public network, fit
his daily behaviour perfectly and gave Iris a new way to make sense of
his "dramatic collapses" and apathy: he had PTSD.

Later on, this recognition of a match between a husband's daily
behaviour and the diagnostic category of PTSD served as a basis for
reorganizing marital relations. Ayala's story provided both therapists
and participants an opportunity to articulate this interpretation. Ayala
is forty-eight-years-old, married to David and a mother of four sons
aged eleven to nineteen. David served as an officer in the Forensic
Science Department of the Israel Police. During the Second Intifada,
he was involved in collecting and identifying body parts from the
sites of terrorist attacks; eventually he was diagnosed with PTSD. The
effects of his symptoms on their marital relations were dramatic, as
Ayala described:

> AYALA: I haven't had marital relations for the last year, and now I've
> made my peace with the situation … It was hard to accept. I thought
> about divorce, but I have stayed with him … Now we sleep in separate
> bedrooms … He had been everything to me: my father and mother, my
> beloved, my husband, my lover, everything … I don't want to brag, but
> he used to behave like a dog in heat. He used to run after me twenty-four
> hours a day, a steed, a bull, and suddenly nothing! Nothing!

SOPHIE (ANOTHER PARTICIPANT): That's the marital relationship, and we do sacrifice. It's a painful acceptance that you bear for the rest of your life.

DINA (THE THERAPIST): It is called compassion ... There is a problem with intimacy. You are all young women. Your physical needs are clear ... Ayala said that she is holding the family together, because even with regard to the children, to simply pick up and leave ...

SOPHIE: That is impossible.

RUTH (ANOTHER PARTICIPANT): We keep saying that we do what we do for him, for the household, and the children. [But] why doesn't anyone ever ask, any month, any week, what is going on with you?!

AYALA (loudly): He is sick! (27 May 2007, Field Notes)

As Ayala's story shows, both the therapist and the participants explicitly expressed what was perceived to be the "appropriate" interpretation of the husband's mental condition. Before being diagnosed with PTSD, David fulfilled every social and romantic function for Ayala: father, mother, beloved, husband, and lover. Not by accident, this holistic description relies on his complete domination over her body. By referring to David's behaviour towards her in animal terms ("a steed," "a bull"), Ayala indirectly validated his masculine identity. The dramatic decline in all these functions because of the disorder prompted her to reformulate their relationship from one of intense physical love ("he used to run after me twenty-four hours a day") to one of caring for a sick spouse.

One of the therapists and a participant presented this restructuring process, which inevitably entailed emphasizing the value of commitment over bodily desire and caring over physical intimacy, as the key mechanism for coping with the man's disorder. Despite their "clear needs" as "young women," they were expected to accept the lack of sexual relations and express compassion while continuing to hold the family together. When Ruth pointed out the inherent inequality of this practice, the profound significance of using medical terms to help understand her husband's suffering became even clearer: "He is sick!" Ayala shouted at her.

A Clinical Definition of Her Own:
"The wife also has to come out of the closet"

Understanding the match between the spouse's daily behaviour and the diagnostic category of PTSD was a preliminary step towards another one: creating a match between the women's condition and the diagnostic category of secondary trauma. An example of this insightful process is found in the story of Iris, mentioned just above. During one of the group sessions, Iris described the acute inequality that developed between her and Yariv after he was diagnosed with PTSD:

> IRIS: He has a privilege. When he doesn't feel well, he goes to sleep ...
> I don't have the privilege to say "I'm shell-shocked." "I'm a second
> generation [Holocaust survivor]." It seems to me that every time he
> thinks I want to talk with him, he gets depressed.
>
> DINA (ONE OF THE THERAPISTS): Stand firm, tell him, "Sit here, I want
> to talk with you!"
>
> IRIS: He just doesn't hear me!
>
> DINA: Do you feel guilty?
>
> IRIS: No, my problem is that I don't talk to him about these kinds of things
> ... I'm the one who listens.
>
> DINA: How do you feel now, when you do talk?
>
> IRIS: That is what I need to do.
>
> DINA: The wife also has to come out of the closet, not just the husband.
>
> AVIVA (ANOTHER PARTICIPANT): The woman's place has been pushed
> completely out of sight. The time is ripe now in society to bring it out.
>
> LIN (THE SECOND THERAPIST): The very fact that you are here today
> is a sign that [society] recognizes that women suffer from secondary
> trauma ... I congratulate you, Iris, on your ability to claim your right
> to your own place. (25 February 2007, Field Notes)

This dialogue between Iris and Aviva (participants) and Dina and Lin (therapists) demonstrates how the men's diagnosis of PTSD extends into the women's diagnosis of secondary trauma. However, the meaning of that process was not only medical. Iris's transition from a "listener" to a "speaker" marked a turning point in redefining her social identity as a victim of trauma. This was accompanied by critical semantic expressions from the therapists ("to come out of the closet" and "[the] ability to claim your right to your own place"), as well as from the participants ("The time is ripe now in society to bring it out"). Furthermore, Iris's new status as a secondary victim of trauma was not just a clinical consequence of her spouse's disorder but also appeared to be a social response to the gender inequity that had developed between them. In the face of Yariv's "privilege" as a PTSD victim ("when he doesn't feel well, he goes to sleep"), Iris claimed a "privilege" of her own: not as a "shell-shocked" or "second generation [Holocaust survivor]," as she sarcastically put it, but as a victim of secondary trauma. Later on, it is suggested that this new position might help her achieve what she had failed to achieve up to now: to stand up to Yariv and say, "Sit here, I want to talk with you!"

The Path of Preservation: "It's as if I grew from the pain"

As the participants gained familiarity with the diagnostic categories of PTSD and secondary trauma, they found various ways to use them in their everyday lives. One dominant application was to juxtapose the two traumatic labels in order to preserve the marital relationship, while reorganizing its basic components, such as love, sexual intimacy, and friendship. An example of this process is the story of Michal. Unlike Ayala, Michal was at the beginning of her married life: thirty-eight years old, mother of two young girls ages four and seven, and married to Ofer for nine years. Ofer worked as an ambulance driver and was diagnosed with PTSD in 2001 after taking part in the evacuation of the dead and wounded from a disco in Tel Aviv after a terror attack. "Ofer picked up everything possible from the terror attacks. He collected all the parts of all the victims, and broke up the family," said Michal at one of the sessions (28 January 2007). However, six months after the group started, Michal sounded quite different:

> Today I'm much more; I can put my finger on what I feel. I feel myself ... I'm going through a process that I don't know if I'll ever get through. Suddenly, I'm growing up! ... I read books about PTSD, and a supportive family is one of the most important things ... [One difficult morning] I called a friend and asked for a hug, because I don't get any from Ofer. These are my choices and I am paying for them. (10 June 2007, Field Notes)

Like Ayala, Michal used the clinical label of PTSD as a means to reorganize her marital life. Her familiarity with the empirical findings that point to the importance of supporting the spouse served as a tool for her when she tried to adapt her daily behaviour to the recommendations in the clinical literature. However, unlike Ayala, Michal also reconstructed her own identity through the clinical label of secondary trauma, and by doing so, actualized the symbolic potential of this process that was evident in Iris's story. Based on Michal's position as a victim of secondary trauma, she described how she had started to relate to herself as an autonomic subject, with a new degree of self-awareness and with the possibility of choice even under constrained circumstances.

The Path of Criticism: "I deserve something too!"

In addition to preservation, some of the participants applied the diagnostic categories of trauma and PTSD for the sake of criticizing the therapists' conservative approach, and even more important, to undermine their marital relations. An example of this process appeared towards the end of the sessions. Lin, the therapist, asked each participant to give artistic expression to the concept of "separation." Hanna, a fifty-five-year-old mother of four adult daughters, created two figures from flexible metal wires, one blue and the other pink. The figures, facing each other and connected by a polyurethane cup, symbolized her relationship with Yaakov, her spouse of over thirty years who was suffering from PTSD after two shooting incidents in a West Bank settlement where they lived. Hanna explained that in the past, her marital relationship with Yaakov had been "very stable and strong," but today, "we hardly have a relationship." Lin interpreted Hanna's work as expressing a desire "to hold Yaakov's hand. Go home," she said, "maybe there is a hand waiting for you." Suddenly, Sophie, one of the participants, interrupted the therapist and cried out:

> SOPHIE: Hanna, you are too horny!
> HANNA: What horny, what are you talking about? I'm telling you there are no marital relations!
> LIN (THERAPIST): The difference between the two figures is that one has a hand, whether on purpose or not. It's a male figure. Perhaps it's a wish.
> ...
> SOPHIE: But he can't get it up, he can't! (All the women and the therapists burst into laughter) (13 July 2008, Field Notes)

The terms Sophie used in response to Hanna's work constituted an alternative interpretation to the one suggested by the therapist. In the face of the attempt to see Hanna's work as an expression of her desire to hold Yaakov's hand, Sophie turned the attention to her sexual needs. While clinical studies frequently relate to the decline of physical intimacy with non-judgmental terms, such as "low libido" or "decline in sexual functioning" (cf. Dekel et al., 2005; Jordan et al., 1992; Monson, Taft, and Fredman, 2009; Sayers et al., 2009), Sophie used vulgar expressions ("horny," "he can't get it up") to deliver a much cruder and pithier description of their marital relations.

The deconstructing potential embedded in this alternative interpretation became clear with the story of Dalit, married to Tamir and a mother of four adult children, who was referred to at the beginning of this chapter. Tamir, Dalit's husband, got caught up in a terrorist attack at a shopping mall in the centre of Israel in November 2002, and a few months later, he was diagnosed with PTSD. Soon afterward, he lost his job as a result of severe outbursts of rage. At the beginning of the group sessions, the therapists recommended that Dalit meet with NATAL's psychiatrist who advised her to take antidepressants. A few months later, however, she informed the therapists:

> I am not taking the medicine. It doesn't change the reality, and it only gets worse ... It hurts me, and I want it to hurt ... Officials suddenly showed up with a foreclosure order because we didn't pay some debts! And they even wrote [on the order] that out of consideration they didn't break into the house, and that was lucky because I would have killed myself right in front of them! If you [her husband] love me so much, why are you murdering me this way?! (25 February 2007, Field Notes)

In her refusal to take the antidepressants, Dalit rebelled against her new status as a "patient." Like Luz, the Chilean victim of domestic violence who claimed that the sedatives she received were only "a way not to suffer, not to feel" (Parson, 2010: 73), Dalit felt the medication forced her into passive acceptance of an insufferable reality. She pointed out the financial consequences of her husband's disorder that led to unemployment, debts, and possible loss of their home. Then, she expressed a symbolic threat of death, by suicide ("I would have killed myself") or by her husband ("Why are you murdering me this way?"). The reaction from one of the therapists was of particular interest:

> Within your life of no choice, you still have the possibility of the medication ... It doesn't change the reality, but it can improve your mood so that the reality will be more bearable. The choice is in your hands regarding this small things ... Listen to the psychiatrist, from tonight take the dose he prescribed for you. (25 February 2007, Field Notes)

The therapist, as it turned out, limited Dalit's options to taking the antidepressant or not, while encouraging her to choose the former in order to improve her mood and avoid pain. Though the clinical and domestic contexts differ from those of Ayala and Michal, once again the gendered ideology guiding the group sessions from the therapist's point of view became clear: Lin was indirectly asking Dalit to preserve her marriage despite the severe difficulties it entailed.

Dalit did start taking the antidepressants again. However, it soon became clear that her protest against her position as "patient" was only a preliminary step towards a much more intense protest against her husband. A few months after her declaration regarding the medicine, she stated her intention of leaving her husband, the quotation with which the chapter opens: "I am trying to see how I can extricate myself from this marriage, how to say goodbye." After Dalit's remarks, the room became absolutely still. In other cases of women married to men diagnosed with PTSD, they usually avoided even talking about the option of divorce (see Dekel et al., 2005). This was the first time one of the participants had explicitly expressed such an intention. Like Sophie in her interpretation of Hanna's work, Dalit also emphasized sexual desire, but in opposition to those advocating adherence to the conservative path: the more Tamir tried to get intimate with her, the more she rejected him ("For half a year already, I haven't slept next to him"). Dina, one of the therapists, was the first to respond:

DINA: The question is the children ... You will always remain their mother and he will always remain their father, no matter what his level of functioning.

LIN (THE SECOND THERAPIST): You must make another effort before you start making announcements ... You can make a new [marital] contract ... Leaving is always an option.

IRIS (suddenly bursts out): That's not true! It's not so easy to leave. You need strength for that too. It's not always possible.

DALIT: Sometimes I have the feeling that no one can really understand us, not even you [the therapists].

IRIS: I also feel such self-negation, like I'm nothing ... Why do I have to be this way? Enough, enough! I deserve better than this, I do! And she does too!

DINA (THERAPIST): You don't have to stay together at all cost, but think about the children; they are the victims.

DALIT: Maybe the National Insurance Institute [Social Security] should have explained to all the trauma casualties how to maintain their marital relations.

IRIS (ironically): The National Insurance Institute will do that just like the Rehabilitation Department of the Ministry of Defense actually rehabilitates anyone! Listen, I told Dalit about an apartment for rent for only $200. That is a doable financial option. We can live there together (smiling at Dalit).

RUTH: Can I join too?

LAURIE: We'll set up a women's commune there. (14 October 2007, Field Notes)

Dalit's stated intention of leaving her husband demonstrated how the participation in the group actually equipped her with tools to articulate the possibility of divorce. The familiarity she acquired with the two diagnostic categories, PTSD and secondary trauma, which was supposed to help her reorganize her marital relations with Tamir, led her precisely in the opposite direction, prompting her to draw a new boundary between them. Understanding Tamir's uncontrollable behaviour allowed her to base her frustration on a clinical, thus highly recognized, model. This particular use of the psychiatric definition became even more intense when Dalit used medical terms to help explain her situation, describing herself as suffering from ongoing mental problems ("I take sleeping pills because he infuriates me, he makes me crazy").

At that point, Iris chimed in, and together with Dalit protested against the inferior position assigned to them in both the clinical and social arenas. Iris and Dalit challenged the therapists' professional authority when they criticized Dina's and Lin's conservative reaction to Dalit's decision, immediately invoking the women's ultimate role as mother. Dalit and Iris insisted on the option of taking care of themselves first, in order to defy the clinical and social priority given to the men ("Enough, enough! I deserve better than this, I do!"). This reconstruction of their social identity through "shifting meanings" (Parson, 2010: 79) was fortified by referring to the broader social context: the incompetence of state agencies, such as the National Insurance Institute and the Ministry of Defense, in treating trauma victims and their families. Ruth's and Laurie's support, by asking to live together with Dalit and Iris, demonstrated the potential empowerment offered by the social support of a women's network (Parson, 2010; Warner, 2007).

In the end, Dalit did not divorce Tamir. At the next meeting, she explained she could not muster the courage to leave him. But the possibility had been articulated and paved the way: a few months later, it was

Iris who declared her intention of leaving Yariv. Unlike Dalit, she went through with it. She now lives with her three children in an apartment that costs $200 a month. The rent has probably gone up since then, but Iris still lives there. Two years ago, she remarried.

Conclusion

In this chapter, I have shed light on the first extension of the iconic definition of PTSD towards a subdefinition of secondary trauma. This process created a new circle of negotiation around mental suffering, between the primary diagnostic category of PTSD and secondary trauma, and between clinical concerns and sociopolitical dynamics. These all swirled around between the man and the woman, and between the kitchen and the bedroom, with each definition affecting the other.

Consistent with the contemporary clinical literature (see Dekel et al., 2005; Jordan et al., 1992; Milliken et al., 2007; Sayers et al., 2009; Solomon et al., 2008), the group sessions were meant to help the Israeli women develop skills to cope with their spouses' symptoms, while avoiding secondary traumatic symptoms themselves. However, this clinical agenda met head-on with the particular local context of Israel. In this context, the explanation of trauma and PTSD by mental health experts was tied to a military orientation and sociocultural gender roles (Bilu and Witztum, 2000; Lomsky-Feder, 2004). Although the therapists perceived the group sessions as based on neutral clinical concerns, it turned out that the meetings merged psychiatric labels with gender dynamics and became a site of negotiations. Within this unintended expansion of the group's original mandate, the women have tried to redefine their position as victims of secondary trauma vis-à-vis their spouses' diagnoses of PTSD, while addressing governmental agencies like the Ministry of Defense and the National Insurance Institute.

From the start, NATAL established the group based on the assumption that the medical diagnoses of the men should be expanded to apply to their wives. However, it soon became clear that this presumably neutral process took on another meaning: under the political circumstances of Israel, the women's distress was subordinated to the men's, in both clinical and sociocultural senses. On the one hand, the recognition of the men's suffering was based on using the medical diagnostic category of PTSD. Like the residents of Haiti (James, 2004), Bali (Dwyer and Santikarma, 2007), Liberia (Abramowitz, 2010), and the Mayan refugees in Mexico (Warner, 2007), the position of the Israeli men was articulated through the scientific, highly legitimate status as victims of trauma assigned to them by the official mental health institutions of Israel.

The women's distress, on the other hand, entitled them to a less comprehensive process for using medical terms to understand their experience. The main social site in which the category of secondary trauma could be invoked and examined in relation to the women's condition was during the group sessions. This occurred either by the therapists (as when Iris described Yariv's misuse of his PTSD diagnosis and the therapists pointed out she was suffering from secondary trauma), or by the participants themselves (as when Dalit declared that her spouse's behaviour was driving her "crazy"). The women's distress, thus, was left dangling between the expertise of the therapists, the sociocultural meaning attributed to prolonged violent conflict, and their traditional roles as caregivers within the family. Because they lacked the official stamp of the mental health authorities as secondary trauma victims, understanding their situation as secondary trauma victims turned out to be much more partial, selective, and vague compared to the one associated with the men.

This inequality between the men's and women's clinical framings was also related to the etiology of trauma. The source of the men's trauma dovetailed precisely with the iconic definition of PTSD (see Young, 1995) – a singular event occurring during military service or while being exposed to a terror attack – that Israeli state agencies had already identified as a legitimate cause of trauma. At the same time, the women experienced distress in a much more private, more secretive site of social interaction: marital relations. Although the relationship between trauma and women's everyday experiences has already been examined – Chilean women suffering from ongoing domestic violence (Parson, 2010) and Guatemalan Mayan women in southern Mexico (Warner, 2007) – here it became clear how the primary and well-recognized cause of men's trauma unfolded into routine family life and threatened women's sense of security and stability. Yet the women's painful experiences had much vaguer and more elusive qualities, and therefore, were less intense and persuasive than the ones identified with the men.

As seen throughout this chapter, the relative prioritization between the traumatic injuries of the men versus their spouses was embedded in the Israeli family institution. From the beginning, men's trauma was identified with the dominant Zionist ethos of heroism (Kimmerling, 1993). The Israeli society perceived serving in the IDF or police force to be the ultimate expression of masculinity: active participation in the effort to maintain the strength of the nation (Lieblich, 1978; Lomsky-Feder, 2004). Although public attention regarding PTSD in men was a new manifestation of this ideal (Bilu and Witztum, 2000), in many ways it was but another expression of male "virtue." In face of this newly revealed weakness of the male psyche, the women were expected to more fervently fulfil their traditional role as caregiver, similar to giving birth and raising children (Herzog, 1999; Moore, 2012; Sachs, Sa'ar, and Aharoni, 2007).

Within this deep interconnection between mental health expertise, national conflict and the family, the therapists almost took it for granted that the participants should make every effort to maintain their marriages and continue to hold the family together. Like war widows in Israel, who were perceived first and foremost as the human carriers of their husbands' memory (Shamgar-Handelman, 1986), these women also faced a strong expectation to stay with their spouses despite the dramatic change in their marital relations.

However, despite the restrictive conditions imposed on them in both the clinical and sociocultural arenas, the women in the group tended to analyse quite differently their self-identities within their marriages. Even the partial use of medical information to understand their distress served as an important source of legitimacy for all of them to carry out a profound process of self-reflection. Like the Chilean women engaged in group therapy via an international NGO (Parson, 2010), the Israeli women also redefined their position as embedded within a communal framework, comparing what it had been to what it had become and what it could be. Furthermore, using a more fluid process for translating the participants' mental distress into a subdefinition of trauma, changed the position of the group's therapists. Unlike the interventions carried out in non-Western areas, the therapists were not exclusive "brokers of trauma" (James, 2004: 140). Instead, the participants, who shared similar national and feminine identities with the therapists, felt close enough to the therapists to challenge their privileged status as trauma experts. This critical standpoint allowed the participants to negotiate their marital relations in a creative and impromptu manner, uncovering the diverse ways in which they understood and implemented the two psychiatric labels vis-à-vis their husbands' diagnoses as PTSD victims and their potential diagnoses as secondary trauma victims. Most of them (like Ayala and Michal) used the familiarity they acquired with both clinical concepts to reorganize their traditional role as caregiver and to maintain their marriage. Others, like Iris and Dalit, used it in order to underscore a boundary they felt had grown between them and their spouses, and to express criticism of state agencies.

In the next chapter, I present a further distancing from the clinical nucleus of PTSD through an ethnographic examination of the politics that evolved around therapeutic interventions among diverse ethnonational "at-risk groups."

Chapter Six

Wandering PTSD: Ethnic Diversity and At-Risk Groups across the Country

One day a friend [whose son was killed in the First Lebanon War] calls me and says, "I need to talk to you." We set up a meeting. He asks, "Tell me, what is going to happen to me and my wife?" I looked at him and spoke words. He got up, bent down to me, and said, "Farkash, kiss my ass. I didn't call you here to sell me words. I called you so you would tell me what's going to happen to me and my wife." I looked at him and said, "If you think that time will pass and you'll get free of [your son], you're wrong. Don't think like that. It's not going to happen. He'll be with you when you get up in the morning, when you drink coffee, when you start the car. He'll come at you from the window on the right, drop down in front of your eyes, say to you 'Hi, Dad.' When you return home he'll come at you from the left, 'Hi, Dad.' Wherever you go and whatever you do, he'll be with you." … The [treatment] of bereavement – any trick, any arrangement, it seems to me, like people say – is a sheer waste of time. I coped with it in my own way, and there are no criteria.

– David Farkash, speaking at a seminar for bereaved parents, 19 July 2005

This description by David Farkash, a bereaved father who lost his son in the Yom Kippur War of 1973, marks the migration of trauma and PTSD from the confines of the individual patient–therapist relationship within the clinic, out to the larger community of "at-risk groups." Like PTSD and secondary trauma, the extension of the professional treatment of mental vulnerability beyond the disorder's clinical nucleus towards at-risk groups has also come under critical examination. While epidemiologists may contend that being "at risk" is a single, clear-cut mental state, the concept carries multiple meanings. Being at risk is traditionally understood as indirect exposure to traumatic events through physical closeness to certain threats, or through family relatives and the media, as in the case of the September 11 attacks (Silver et al., 2002). However, it has become evident that exposure to existential threats may have different mental effects across different social populations due to diverse sociopolitical factors. A recent study in Afghanistan, to take only one example, led researchers to claim that social exclusion dynamics that were already in place before the conflict influenced both mental vulnerability during the war and patterns of recovery after the war (Trani and Bakshi, 2013).

As can be seen by Farkash's remarks, this extension towards larger and more diverse groups has made the definition of trauma more familiar and accessible, but at the same time it has provoked criticism and resistance. Like his friend who lost his son in the First Lebanon War in 1982, Farkash was also a secular Ashkenazi Jew whose parents came to Israel from Eastern Europe in the early 1930s. Over the years, Farkash absorbed the local militaristic orientation of Israel after its establishment as an independent Jewish state (Bilu and Witztum, 2000; Kimmerling, 1993; Shafir and Peled, 2002). From this particular point of view, he deemed mental assistance with the pain of loss to be unnecessary. Farkash explained that the son's figure would always accompany the father, while he was drinking coffee or starting the car, and nothing would ever change that. Having depicted this symbiosis between the living father and the departed son, Farkash plainly asked the trauma experts not "to sell words," because it's "a sheer waste of time. I coped with it in my own way, and there are no criteria."

In this chapter, thus, I trace the branching out of trauma from its clinical home base to four at-risk groups in Israel, each representing a different ethno-national context established in Israel alongside the secular Ashkenazi group. The first one involves a group of National Orthodox Jewish mentors from Ezer me-Tzion, an NGO in the ultra-Orthodox city of Bnei Brak. These mentors accompanied children living in Jewish settlements in the Occupied Territories (especially in the Gaza Strip and the northern West Bank) whose families had suffered harm in terror attacks (August–September 2005). The second context entails a group of female Bedouin social workers who treated patients suffering from mental, as well as physical, trauma in a large hospital in the southern city of Beer Sheva (January 2006). The third context focuses on a group of bereaved Druze parents who, together with bereaved Jewish parents (like Farkash), participated in a seminar at the Memorial Center in their town, Dalyat el-Carmel (July 2005). Lastly, the fourth context revolves around psychosocial intervention workshops for secular Jewish children from Kibbutz Zikkim, which is adjacent to the Gaza Strip and had been exposed to Qassam rocket fire (February–April 2006). While presenting the mental assistance and patterns of interpretations offered by the mental health experts, special attention will be provided to the participants' repertoire of responses derived from their particular world views. Based on this juxtaposition, I analyse how the local experts made the distinction between traumatic symptoms and other emotional experiences of loss and distress, or perhaps blurred it, while extending their scope of activity into new, sometimes unusual, areas of professional engagement. Under these new circumstances of therapeutic communication, some political, ethnic, and moral issues have been highlighted by both aid providers and aid receivers.

In the Centre: Workshops for National Orthodox Jewish Mentors from Ezer Mizion

The first therapeutic intervention took place within the framework of a project operated by Ezer Mizion. Ezer Mizion is an NGO established in the late 1970s by an ultra-Orthodox Jew, a graduate of one of the large yeshivas in the ultra-Orthodox city of Bnei Brak. Since its establishment, this aid agency has offered paramedical services to assist the ill, disabled, elderly, and other needy groups in Israel. In that spirit, in the summer of 2004 the NGO launched a new project under the slogan "A helping mentoring hand." The purpose was to provide psychosocial support to children living in the settlements of the Gaza Strip and the northern West Bank whose families had suffered harm in terrorist attacks. The young yeshiva students who provided the support, most of them in their twenties, were living in the same settlements.

About a year after the project began, Ezer Mizion leaders initiated therapeutic intervention for the mentors to help them contend with the traumatic circumstances with which the families were coping. At their first meeting, in the opening conversation between the clinical psychologist from NATAL and the yeshiva mentors, the complexity of the weekly encounters between mentor and child quickly became evident. Abraham, for example, a yeshiva student from the Jewish settlement of Kedumim, related, "The boy's father was badly injured in a shooting attack … The boy tells me that in his dreams he dreams that something is trying to catch and eat him, and he's trying to escape." He explained his willingness to participate in the work-shop was due to the fact that "practically speaking, we're missing the tools. We haven't learned enough." Another mentor introduced himself as follows: "Amitzur, I study at the yeshiva in [the Jewish settlement of] Itamar. I mentor a boy from the first grade in Itamar whose father was killed." A third mentor, Dvir, who also lived in Kedumim, said he would come to the workshop because "to me it was hard [dealing] with this matter of a child who is undergoing trauma from terror. His mother and three brothers were murdered, and the boy is very withdrawn" (6 July 2005, Field Notes).

Some professional guidance indeed seemed necessary against the background of the traumatic reality characterizing the lives of the children that the yeshiva students were mentoring. Nonetheless, the series of meetings between the mentors and the psychologist were far from merely functional. Another dimension added to the initial ten-sion between the clinical logic underlying trauma discourse and deep religious faith: the meetings took place in the summer months of 2005. Fierce political debate raging at the time over the Disengagement Plan, scheduled to occur at summer's end (discussed in chapter 1), exacerbated the Israeli heat of July and August. Vehement opposi-tion to the implementation of the plan on the part of the participants, many of them residents of those Jewish settlements that were to be evacuated, percolated into the meetings. At times, this conflict cast an unexpected light on the dialogue between the participants and the psychologist, Dr. Levin, a secular Jewish resident of Tel Aviv based in the centre of Israel, whom they identified, and rightfully so, with the left wing in Israel.

From Speech to Action: "The boy says to me,
'This prime minister should have sixty nails
hammered into his head.' What am I supposed to say?"

One of the important principles taught to the mentors in the workshop was empathic communication. Levin, the psychologist, opened one of the meetings by explaining the value of using this form of communica-tion to help children cope with traumatic injury, "It's important to be able to reflect to someone else the emotions evoked by their remarks, without judging them … You reflect the problem, perform validation and justify, even if you do not accept the position" (6 July 2005, Field Notes). After some role-play conducted by the psychologist and one of the mentors, in the course of which they reconstructed an argument between that mentor and his wife, another mentor, Dvir, threw down the gauntlet, "What about the Disengagement Plan?" Levin immediately rose to the challenge, "The Disengagement is a wonderful example. Let's do it. It's a fantastic exercise." The psychologist first represented the supporters of the Disengagement, while Dvir expressed his original stance, opposition, but was required to engage in "empathic communication" with the supporter. Levin opened the exchange:

PSYCHOLOGIST: It's very important for the country [of Israel] that we disengage, that we give peace a chance at last.

DVIR: If I understand you, you think the Palestinians should be given a state.

PSYCHOLOGIST (correcting Dvir's mistake in following the guidelines of empathy): No, try to explain why my position isn't warped.

DVIR (trying again): I understand that you look at the Intifada, at everything they've done, and that they simply must be given a state, because there is no such thing as being able to rule another nation.

PSYCHOLOGIST (smiling broadly): Aha! What an effort! Look how he's sweating! (All laugh) The idea is that you don't have to agree with him, but you mustn't think he's crazy. Let's switch.

The discussion continued as follows, with Levin now in the position of the "empathic listener":

DVIR: I can't understand how you can evict Jews from their homes.

PSYCHOLOGIST: You say you think that the removal of Jews is eviction, because when you think that I, a countryman of yours, am taking you from the place where you have settled, that is eviction. When I speak to you in this way, we meet. If I understand your emotions, then there is a chance that contact is made ... I identify with the emotional side, not with the [political] position but with the emotion behind the matter, and that takes you to a deeper place of understanding.

YEDIDYA (ANOTHER MENTOR, WHO LIKE THE OTHERS HAS BEEN LISTENING ATTENTIVELY): But when you accept, you acknowledge the guilt. That's seemingly how it's perceived.

PSYCHOLOGIST: No, I really think it's an attempt to understand.

YEDIDYA: No, but regarding the Disengagement as you spoke, it's a kind of argument, so it's as if I am with you, but actually ... yes, in feeling [between couples], but in the [context of the] Disengagement [Plan]?

PSYCHOLOGIST: Look, in arguments, there is no absolute justice, [but] if each one understands the other; it's not that each one is entirely either right or wrong ... When you work with children, you don't want to get stuck in a conflict situation.

DVIR (more relaxed, no longer required to engage in empathic communication): But if the boy is angry, so you don't really understand, you don't really think he's right, and at some point it's bound to come out.

PSYCHOLOGIST: Empathy, it's an important stance in life. It's unimportant whether [the situation] is political or emotional. Part of the conflict is that people don't hear each other at all.

YISHAI (ANOTHER MENTOR): But there are arguments that have to be decided!

PSYCHOLOGIST: But there's a chance you'll reach a compromise. There's a chance we'll get to the "grey area," and won't say black and white all the time.

YISHAI: But sometimes the boy I'm mentoring says to me, "This prime minister should have his head chopped off! Bring him to me now, and I will hammer sixty nails into his head." What am I supposed to say? That's right, I understand you, he should have nails stuck in his eye?!

PSYCHOLOGIST: No, you tell him I can understand why you're angry, but you know killing is forbidden ... Be assertive. You don't agree, but you can understand the desire and the anger, and say that even though the anger can lead to things, it need be remembered that killing is forbidden. (6 July 2005, Field Notes)

By using the tool of empathy, the psychologist sought to present guidelines for "correct" communication: how to listen and how to speak. These guidelines reflect the neutral perspective on interactions that characterize the therapeutic discourse (see Illouz, 2008): each party is a subject with emotions and capable, as such, of acknowledging the emotions of the other party. Almost by itself, this approach pushes sociopolitical and class hierarchies into a subordinate position. Instead, the emotional balance between the parties and reaching a mutual avoidance of judgment is the overriding goal.

However, the mentors were in no hurry to accept the guidelines for empathy and the moral assumptions underlying them. Although they regarded them as fairly effective in interpersonal relations (as expressed when one of them agreed to exercise the guidelines for empathy in reenacting an argument with his wife), they were dubious about the effectiveness of shifting this psychological technique from the private to the public sphere of politics. Perceiving actual decision making as based on a rational choice between concrete policy alternatives, the mentors expressed the opinion that this psychological approach was unsuitable for the public sphere. Dvir, who practised empathic communication with the psychologist regarding the Disengagement Plan, found it difficult to implement the guidelines. He did not reflect the emotions of the speaker facing him but rather exposed the political stance implied by his remarks.

This tension between the therapeutic goal – being engaged in empathic communication – and the divided political reality in Israel came close to absurdity. One of the participants, Yishai, wondered how it was possible to engage in empathic communication in the face of the violence that the boy he was mentoring had proposed meting out to the prime minister. In light of the traumatic collective memory of the political assassination of Prime Minister Yitzhak Rabin in November 1995, Yishai asked, "What am I supposed to say? That's right, I understand you, he should have nails stuck in his eye?!" This disparaging example of empathic communication exposed how the avoidance of moral judgment illuminated its moral and practical limitations in relation to controversial political situations that frequently arose in Israel.

In the South: Workshops for Bedouin Social Workers in a Beer Sheva Hospital

In January 2006, NATAL conducted a therapeutic intervention at a large hospital in the southern city of Beer Sheva for female Bedouin social workers. These social workers were assisting patients suffering from mental stress due to terrorist or shooting incidents. The goal of the intervention was to improve the social workers' skills during their interactions with these patients and their family members. Although the hospital's senior staff and the participants themselves perceived their involvement at the meetings as perfectly natural, in Israel's divided demographic reality, their presence has carried a unique meaning. All the social workers belonged to the ethnic and religious minority of the Bedouin community in the Negev that, according to official publications, constitutes a population of about 200,000. Like half of the Bedouin community living in this area, the social workers were residents of the permanent Bedouin town of Rahat in the Negev

Desert.[1] Their work in the hospital, including their participation in the workshop sessions, reflected the changes that have occurred among the women of the Bedouin community over the past two decades. As part of a broader social process, some of them have begun acquiring an academic education, while manoeuvring cautiously between the desire to fulfil traditional gender roles and their longing to blaze a trail and break through the community's boundaries (Abu Rabia-Queder, 2008). The social workers who participated in the workshop certainly brought to it their careful ways of negotiating between working at home and working with professional principals. At home, they were involved in treating members of their community suffering from mental stress, and under the professional principals, they sought to improve their social work skills.

From the Universal to the Particular:
"He might even hit me if I tell him"

At one of the workshop sessions, the Jewish psychologist conducting them, Judith Alon, presented to the social workers the practice of "relaxation." Since it allows practitioners to connect to their inner world, the psychologist described the use of this practice as essential for the purpose of dredging up and processing traumatic experiences. Immediately after the social workers practised this technique, Alon asked to hear whether they found it effective for their work at the hospital. Jamila and Nada were the first to respond:

JAMILA: It [the relaxation] is something that is not connected, something they'll think that I … I don't know. In the Bedouin community – I understand the technique, but I myself don't do relaxation.
NADA: You [the psychologist] have to provide [us] other artistic means, because there are populations that resemble the Bedouin population, even in Israeli society, which refuse to do relaxation.
PSYCHOLOGIST: There are many degrees and levels of relaxation, but the keyword is that there isn't anybody who can't do relaxation; the only

---

1 According to official publications, some 200,000 to 210,000 Bedouin live in the Negev Desert in the south of Israel. Over half reside in seven towns built by the government for the Bedouin, and the remainder live in forty-six villages, thirty-five of which are unrecognized and eleven of which were officially recognized a few years ago.

question is how you refer to it ... Research shows that what happens
during relaxation is the brainwaves are lowered to the alpha level. The
emphasis is that when the brain is in the alpha stage, we are at our most
creative level ... I'd like to say to Jamila, who said that it's not suited to
the Bedouin community, first of all, it's not suited to you as a person at
this moment ... Instead of saying it's not suited to the entire Bedouin
community, say it's not suited to me.

NADA: To me it's very comfortable. Personally, it suits me, even at home.
It's fantastic for me, but it doesn't suit the Bedouin community! It just
doesn't work! With [a] Bedouin [man], if I tell [him] to do relaxation,
he might even hit me if I tell him.

PSYCHOLOGIST: It's true that silence, when relaxation is practised in
tandem, acquires an intimate dimension ... You can try calling it by other
names that are culturally correct ... I'll hand it right back to you, if you
can improve on it.

JAMILA: It doesn't mean I haven't got alternatives. I am part of the
community. I treat the anxious, so we go out for a walk, follow the sheep
... But if I were to sit facing someone older than me and tell him to shut
his eyes, he would think that either I have gone crazy or he has gone
crazy.

PSYCHOLOGIST: There is something very natural and basic about
relaxation, like praying, without any psychological words, only
breathing at different intensities, and then all the resistance drops.
(3 January 2006, Field Notes)

This dialogue brought to the surface an essential conflict between the
universal aspiration of the therapeutic engagement with trauma and
a sociocultural component presented by Nada and Jamila. Based on a
particular view deeply embedded in their daily lives, the two of them
pointed out the unsuitability of the practice of relaxation for the
Bedouin community. Gender and intergenerational social hierarchies
prevalent in the community would make relaxation a practice that
could lead to high levels of embarrassment, anger, and insult, even to
the point of violence.

With these remarks, Nada and Jamila threatened to undermine the
legitimacy of the professional intervention and its effectiveness by
questioning the fulfilment of the therapeutic goal articulated by the
psychologist: to teach them how to use relaxation as a tool for processing traumatic experiences. Therefore, in her response to their resistance,
the psychologist sought to frame relaxation as a natural and neutral

practice that "every" person could exercise and benefit from. She explained the physiological value of relaxation and even compared it to the religious practice of praying. Alon was trying to neutralize the cultural context in which the Bedouin social workers had situated their critical arguments and to make their resistance a personal matter: "It's not suited to you as a person at this moment," she said to Jamila. This response to the Bedouin social workers' resistance revealed, once again, cultural differences as well as ethnic and socio-economic dynamics.

In the North: Seminar for Druze Bereaved Parents from Dalyat el-Carmel

In July 2005, NATAL held a seminar for bereaved parents at the Yad la-Banim[2] Memorial Center of Dalyat el-Carmel, a town of another ethno-national minority in Israel, the Druze. Due to the continuing violence surrounding the Arab–Israeli conflict and the involvement of many citizens in military service, bereavement constitutes a central element of public life in Israel (Kimmerling, 1993). However, the fact that NATAL held the seminar in a Druze community made it quite special. Dalyat el-Carmel is a local council in northern Israel with a population of 16,000 residents, and it is the largest demographic concentration of Druze in Israel. According to the history accepted by the Druze community elders, which also appears in official government publications, the Druze settlement in this area began in the first half of the seventeenth century. After Israel's establishment in 1948, the Druze found themselves in a vulnerable civic position. As an ethnic and religious minority in a Jewish state, they were excluded from the national "we" and sometimes were even identified, explicitly and implicitly, as a subversive group (Shafir and Peled, 2002). In 1957, almost a decade after Israel's establishment, the government officially declared the Druze a "religious minority," and since then their men have been required to serve in the military. While Druze women, similar to the Orthodox Jewish women, were exempt from conscription on religious grounds, a military unit for Druze men was established in the IDF, and today it is considered to be one of the

2 The Yad la-Banim organization was established in 1949 as the representative association on behalf of the State of Israel charged with commemorating soldiers killed during their military service. In many Israeli cities and towns, there is a Yad la-Banim Memorial Center that coordinates the organization's activities vis-à-vis the local residents.

best units in the IDF. Furthermore, over the years, the rate of Druze men serving in command positions, as officers or non-commissioned officers, has been significantly higher than their relative percentage in the Israeli population. The result has been the tragic statistics of the many fallen soldiers from within the Druze community, and the intense experience of bereavement trauma among its members. NATAL psychologists, therefore, carried out the seminar within a unique ethno-nationalist context of bereavement and, during the seminar, deep tensions emerged between the therapeutic discourse on PTSD and the Druze's religious faith. This tension highlighted their ongoing ambiguous civic position in Israel, as illustrated in the next section.

From Emotion to Politics: "We're in a Catholic marriage"

Dr. Berger, a clinical psychologist and NATAL senior staff member, opened the seminar with the following statement:

> It's important to us to be here, because in my view the Druze sector, like other minorities in Israel, has not received sufficient resources. I've worked in many communities in Israel ... and we still haven't reached the Druze community, and that's something that needs to be corrected ... I hope this day will blaze the trail. (19 July 2005, Field Notes)

As can be seen, Berger situated the seminar within Israel's divided political context, seeking to present it as a symbolic repair of the ongoing discrimination that the Druze community have been suffering over the years. However, immediately afterwards, Berger went on to explain that the seminar was intended for "people who are stuck in the bereavement process. There is not much talk about it. Ten per cent don't recover, can't function. They need help." Having presented the therapeutic goal, Berger presented to his audience the specific diagnostic category of PTSD resulting from it – "traumatic grief":

> What is traumatic grief? The non-acceptance of death, rage and bitterness over the death of someone, terrible and unceasing pain and sorrow, an inability to enjoy anything pleasurable, persistent memories, primarily of the agonizing death itself ... Ladies and gentlemen, this is problematic bereavement, and we [the mental health experts] think we can treat it at the clinical level; you can get out of it, get your life back and move on. (19 July 2005, Field Notes)

With this description, Berger took a sharp turn in the way he framed the experience of bereavement. From his opening statement regarding the tense political context in which the bereavement occurred, he moved to the neutral clinical framing of the loss through a specific clinical concept – "traumatic grief." By means of this definition, he sought to identify the most vulnerable group among the bereaved parents, those suffering from "problematic bereavement," and to open before them the possibility of mental aid. However, the next speaker after Berger, Amal Nasser a-Din, the chair of the Druze Memorial Center, objected:

> There is no power in the world that can make a bereaved person forget, none. But for the Druze, belief in reincarnation is very helpful to us … No factor can return life to that person, when the hour comes – pauper or king. [But] faith is very strengthening. I'm not saying we don't have feelings – anger, pain – that we all go through. But we know that there is nothing to be done. Therefore, [you should] accept it from God. (19 July 2005, Field Notes)

In his response to Berger's opening argument, Nasser a-Din resorted to religious faith for the sake of contending with bereavement and thereby sought to undermine the proposal to cope with it therapeutically. In contrast to the framing of emotional difficulties presented by Berger through the clinical concept of "traumatic grief," Nasser a-Din posited faith in God and belief in reincarnation as much more effective coping tools to help weave the experience of loss into daily life. Along the way, Nasser a-Din also shed light on what he perceived to be the limitations of any person, including therapists and experts. He explained that however harsh the feelings might be, death was an unchangeable fact, scarcely susceptible to relief or assistance, and therefore we must accept it as such.

The third speaker, a secular Jew, did not share Nasser a-Din's belief in reincarnation, but he also found the therapeutic engagement with bereavement trauma ineffective, even infuriating. His name was Yossi Harari, a bereaved Jewish father and member of the Yad la-Banim national secretariat:

> After the learned lecture [by Dr. Berger], I would like to contradict it slightly from our [the bereaved parents'] position. Bereavement is a personal thing; I can't do averages and generalizations with it … No offense meant, but whoever hasn't undergone [it] can't understand … I've been a

bereaved father for thirty-three years, since the Yom Kippur War [1973], and my wife treats it one way, myself another … I'm not a doctor, and I haven't brought you any surveys. I've brought you problems that I've run into, the solution to which is not mathematical. It's not written in any book … Whoever thinks he's got a mathematical solution for this issue, I think he's mistaken, but let him speak. Every person is a separate soul, with different needs, and you've got to adapt to his needs. (19 July 2005, Field Notes)

Harari undermined the therapeutic approach, not by means of religious faith as Nasser a-Din had done before him but by arguing for the existence of a personal experience of loss. He contended that this experience changed from mother to father and from one person to the next. Therefore, any attempt to quantify it was fundamentally mistaken. From his point of view, the surveys, averages, and generalizations expressed by a clinical concept, such as "traumatic grief," were incapable of giving expression to the uniqueness of bereavement situated deep inside the soul.

In the second part of the seminar, the participants dispersed into small groups, in which they conducted a conversation regarding their daily ability to cope with loss. When the groups finished working, the participants reassembled again in the Memorial Center's main hall. The privilege of concluding the seminar was given to Nasser a-Din, who provided a summary:

In order to study the Druze problem [in Israel] more than a seminar is needed. We are a community. It's important that every Jew know that before 1948 we believed in the way of the Jewish leaders … Our connection with the Jews is not from today, not from one hundred years ago, but since Moses the Lawgiver … It's a sign that we're in the same boat, that we are brethren … As a Druze, although I'm an unadulterated Israeli, I ask that we work together … We are not mercenaries. We do it with love. When the Jews didn't have money, we brought out weapons and money to them from Syria, from Lebanon … The Druze community is the only one in the Middle East that says to the Jews, "We are brothers, not just friends, brothers." I'm a Druze, I'm an Israeli Druze. We don't want to be Arabs. We are not against Arabs. We do not hate human beings … The moment the Arab sends his son to the army, when he willingly raises the Israeli flag, shows that he's an inseparable part [of this country], then I'll be willing to salute him. We're in a Catholic marriage, the Jews and the Druze. (19 July 2005, Field Notes)

Nasser a-Din's final remarks demonstrate how therapeutic engagement with bereavement trauma, "traumatic grief" in the psychologist's terms, intersects with the group's identity and ethno-national politics. Nassar a-Din characterizes the confusing civic position of the Druze in Israeli society as belonging, yet set apart (Shafir and Peled, 2002). He contrasts this to the Arabs, who do not "willingly raise the Israeli flag," but at the same time the Druze have not been entirely assimilated into the Jewish national "we." Nasser a-Din described the long-standing political alliance between the Druze and the Jews as being based on exchanges of money, weapons, and blood. That alliance, he hinted, was of greater standing than the alliance the seminar sought to emphasize: the emotional bond among Druze and Jewish bereaved parents contending with loss in similar circumstances. However, from his point of view the two alliances are not mutually exclusive but rather strengthen one another. Both of them make possible the seemingly impossible mixing of the Druze and Jewish identities: "I'm an Israeli Druze," Nasser-a-Din said about himself, but also "an unadulterated Israeli."

On the Kibbutz: Workshops for Secular Jewish Children from Zikkim

The therapeutic intervention with which I shall conclude this chapter is ostensibly the most crucial one: with the young children of Kibbutz Zikkim. Like many other kibbutzim Israel established along its borders, Kibbutz Zikkim also represents the combination of Zionism and socialism embedded within its unique communal structure (Shafir and Peled, 2002). In 1949, Jewish immigrants from Romania established Zikkim adjacent to the Gaza Strip. In the early years, numerous border incursions exacted a heavy price in lives lost and led to the departure of most of its members, bringing the kibbutz to the brink of dissolution. Jewish immigrants from England arrived there to strengthen the settlement, and beginning in 1967, groups of immigrants from South America joined the kibbutz. Today, 160 members reside in Zikkim, and its economy is based on agricultural crops, a dairy, and a plastics industry.

Since the beginning of the Second Intifada in October 2000, the kibbutz residents have been exposed to Qassam rocket fire from the Gaza Strip. As a result, NATAL conducted therapeutic interventions, especially for the children of the primary school. The goal was to help them emotionally process their prolonged exposure to rocket fire. Dr. Reuven Segev and Yehudit Sharon, two clinical psychologists living in the centre of Israel, came to the kibbutz several times and conducted workshops for the children.

From Individual Difficulties to Communal Correction: "Zikkim is with God!"

In April 2006, the therapeutic intervention for the children assumed a sociodramatic cast. The psychologists divided the children, who had gathered at the kibbutz community centre, into three groups. They asked each group to present a different chapter in the life of the kibbutz: past ("before the time Qassams fell here"), present ("now, when you're coping with the Qassams"), and future ("what will it be like ten, twenty years from now"). After an hour of feverish preparations, during which the children bustled about the club trying on costumes and collecting various props, the show began. The first group to take the improvised stage (a large mat spread over the floor) were the five children portraying the past. Three of them represented the original Jewish settlers in Zikkim, and one girl was dressed in traditional Arab clothing. Another fifth grader, Noi, narrated this part of the show, opening with an explanation:

> NOI: After three months [since immigrating to Israel], we arrived to establish Kibbutz Zikkim, we the Romanians, and we sang the anthem: "The two-thousand-year-old hope; to be a good kibbutz that the Romanians established in our land!"[3]
>
> GALI (THE GIRL WEARING TRADITIONAL ARAB CLOTHING): Allah akbar! Allah akbar! Allah akbar! (She pours tea into cups and serves them to the three other children)
>
> TOMER (A BOY, TO GALI): Thank you, we're done. Can you sit down and talk with us? We want to establish a kibbutz here, a kibbutz of Romanians. Will you let us? In short, we'll give you some money. You're going to Gazuza, and you're giving us the kibbutz and never coming back. See how much money we have? Sign here, to confirm you won't come here anymore! (After the "Arab" girl signs) Take the money and get lost. How wonderful! Now we can establish a kibbutz. (30 April 2006, Field Notes)

---

3 Paraphrasing the Israeli national anthem, "The Hope" (Hatikvah in Hebrew), and especially the following sentences: "The two-thousand-year-old hope. To be a free people in our homeland. The land of Zion and Jerusalem."

The group depicting the present consisted of two girls, Alma and Naama, playing the roles of mothers sitting and discussing the possibility of leaving the kibbutz. A third girl, Tali, who played the role of a counsellor, listened to them. Two boys, Ariel and Tamar, narrated:

TAMAR: Welcome, you've arrived at the present, the period with rocket alarms.

ALMA: I can't take it anymore with the security situation in the kibbutz, Qassams and Palestinians all the time!

NAAMA (sighing): I can't sleep at night either, but we've got to stay here. It's the kibbutz we've always lived in.

(In light of the disagreement between them, the two girls declare their intention of turning to a counsellor who is sitting on the floor)

TALI (THE COUNSELOR): I would like to recommend [the lighting of incense] candles!

NAAMA (angrily): What has that got to do with it? There's a security situation here, Qassams, rocket alarms!

ARIEL (making siren noises): Red dawn! Red dawn! Red dawn![4]

Alma and Naama scurry about looking for shelter, while Tali remains in her place on the floor.

ARIEL: Boom!!!

TALI (her eyes darting about): What was that?

ALMA: A rocket alarm! But the Qassam has already fallen!

TALI (regaining composure): I recommend doing yoga during a rocket attack. Again, I must tell you that lighting candles is the best thing.

ALMA & NAAMA: What's this nonsense? Lighting candles won't help us!

TALI: Presents are the best thing!

(The two girls get up to leave, clearly disappointed with the results of counselling, while the counsellor again remains in her place)

---

4 The official code word for a rocket alarm used by the Israeli early warning system.

TALI: Nonetheless, I recommend lighting candles! (30 April 2006, Field Notes)

In their part of the show, the group performing the future played a family, huddled inside a small room, who are reminded that the next day is their young son's birthday. The segment began with an announcement by one of the boys: "The year is 2017, the Arabs have advanced and they've got atom bombs. We are living in shelters."

MOTHER: What shall we do?
FATHER: We'll take a chance and go out to buy him a present.
MOTHER: Where is Gal [the little boy's sister]?
FATHER: She went to get food.
MOTHER (with grim conviction): She'll blow up, like the building.
GIRL IN THE AUDIENCE: It's as if it's the Holocaust. They've got nothing to eat.
BOY SITTING NEXT TO HER: That's right. It's like the wars there used to be.

(The children concluded the three segments of their show with a rousing rendition of the kibbutz's anthem)

ALL: Oh, Zikkim, how much we love you/Married only to you;
All night and all day/It is only of you we dream;
Oh, Zikkim!/I thank God I'm not from Miflasim,
Not from Karmiya, and not from Nir-Am;[5]
Zikkim, upward and onward!
All kibbutzim are in heaven, but Zikkim is with God! (30 April 2006, Field Notes)

After singing the kibbutz's anthem, the children wanted to give the two psychologists a parting gift: "We'll give Reuven a Qassam and Yehudit a Katyusha."[6]

---

5 Names of other kibbutzim Israel established near Zikkim and adjacent to the Gaza Strip.

6 Katyusha is the name of the missiles fired against northern Israel by the military organization of Hezbollah, operating from the state of Lebanon.

Observing the performance by the kibbutz children, it should be noticed, first, that all of its three scenes, were predominantly characterized by their full control over its content. Besides the general instructions they had been given to divide their presentation into three segments – past, present, and future – not one of the groups asked for any help in the preparations for the show or during its course. The psychologists, Segev and Sharon, quickly became ordinary spectators, their therapeutic knowledge being of no practical significance with respect to what was going on.

This high degree of freedom the children employed in dramatizing the narrative of the kibbutz led to a rowdy spectacle. With no coordination among the groups, they all placed the kibbutz story, including their exposure to Qassam rockets, in a highly political context. Aware of the kibbutz's history, the children characterized the past by the expulsion of the Arabs in exchange for money, and the future by an apocalyptic atmosphere of devastation and self-preservation due to growing Arab power. Along the way the children poked fun at state symbols, such as the national anthem and the ethos of the kibbutz's foundation ("The two-thousand-year-old hope to be a good kibbutz that the Romanians established in our land!").

Regarding the present, the girls of the group expertly situated the relationship between them as aid receivers and the therapists as aid providers within a hierarchical context. The ludicrous character of the counsellor represented the therapists' disconnection from the troubling experience of rocket attacks: the counsellor had never been exposed to rocket fire as evidenced by her having no idea what "Red dawn!" meant. Furthermore, recommending the use of techniques such as yoga and lighting candles was clearly useless in a life-threatening situation, another indication of the disconnection between the counsellor and the people she intended to assist. Another marker of the power dynamic between the therapists and those they were there to treat was the children's choice of parting gifts to the psychologists: to one of them a Qassam and to the other a Katyusha.

Between past, present, and future, the children of Kibbutz Zikkim constructed a political narrative, neither traumatic nor therapeutic. It was a story devoid of any qualities of processing or relief and, instead, was sprinkled with grim messages of termination and extinction. The overall effect was a parodic carnival atmosphere. Within this emotional and social mixture, the most important message was not an individual one but rather a communal one of belonging to the kibbutz: "All kib-butzim are in heaven," sang the children, "but Zikkim is with God!"

Conclusion

In this chapter, I have traced the wanderings of trauma and PTSD through four groups that while being defined as "at risk" were also ethno-nationally diverse. Under the broader term of "at risk," the experts have constantly challenged the conservative boundaries of their professional work. From the Bedouins in the south to the Druze in the north, the experts relied on the high legitimacy attributed to trauma as a clinical concept. However, it was precisely this legitimacy that allowed them to move beyond the nucleus of the disorder and extend their scope of activity to those who had not been diagnosed as suffering from traumatic or post-traumatic symptoms but only as having the potential to develop them.

This mode of therapeutic assistance first emerged in the U.S. following the attacks of September 11. Mental health experts in the U.S. perceived the events as a turning point in how they needed to think about existential threats, and a new professional sensitivity to the uncertainty that characterizes life under the new global threat of terrorism has developed since then (Furedi, 2004; Young, 2007). However, alongside experts' attempts to provide relief and a feeling of security in conflict and disaster areas, these therapeutic interventions have also drawn heavy criticism. Researchers have argued that the professional effort to provide individual-oriented assistance is embedded with the assumption that the lay person has no control over reality around him or her, thus he or she will always be cast in the role of a "helpless victim" (see Pupavac, 2001).

In the Israeli context of prolonged and violent conflict, however, the professional engagement with mental vulnerability among large groups has somehow led to new social arenas. The interweaving of clinical issues – which are perceived to be objective and neutral (treating at-risk groups to prevent post-traumatic symptoms) – with the political dynamic of national belonging (post-traumatic symptoms as a result of political conflict) in many ways has made it possible to deliver the particular viewpoints of the participants through the clinical construct of trauma. It was precisely the professional and apolitical engagement with mental vulnerability that allowed the communal experiences of political dynamics and ethno-national inequalities to be illuminated. This unintended consequence of the therapeutic interventions – far beyond their original, clinical, and neutral goal – gave them their multi-layered quality.

On the one hand, the experts' declared purpose was to offer mental aid (namely, knowledge and tools) for improving coping skills among National Orthodox Jewish mentors of the Ezer Mizion NGO, among Bedouin social workers in the south, among Druze bereaved parents in the north, and among secular Jewish children from Kibbutz Zikkim. On the other hand, this original goal of intervention frequently turned out to produce multiple responses that unravelled gradually as the interventions proceeded. The participants confronted the therapists regarding the mental assistance provided. This unravelling exposed the moral viewpoints, originally embedded in the traumatic experience, that rose to the surface during the interventions.

From these moral viewpoints, the participants frequently argued against the clinical principles guiding the therapeutic intervention with its universal and apolitical qualities. The participants argued against the experts' efforts to classify and categorize their suffering into quantified, fixed definitions (as in the case of the interventions among Druze and Jewish bereaved parents in Dalyat el-Carmel and among Bedouin social workers). The participants' criticisms and resistance sprang from the multitude of prior experiences they brought to the therapeutic meetings. While the Bedouin social workers came with cultural experiences of the gender hierarchy within the Bedouin community, the National Orthodox mentors arrived with political and religious beliefs about the impending evacuation of their homes. While the bereaved Druze parents arrived with political and religious beliefs about their position as an Arab minority in Israel, the children of Kibbutz Zikkim turned up with a historical narrative about the proximity of their community to the Gaza Strip.

Furthermore, the ability to highlight sociopolitical fault lines was thanks to the shared tendency of both aid providers and receivers to perceive the therapeutic discourse as creating a neutral, even sterile environment. It's not about politics but about mental vulnerability. Nevertheless, in the absence of clear diagnosed symptoms, an essential change occurred in the fundamental position of the National Orthodox Jewish mentors from Ezer Mizion, of the Bedouin social workers from Beer Sheva, of the Druze bereaved parents from Dalyat el-Carmel, and of the secular Jewish children from Kibbutz Zikkim. Their position was not that of "patients" but as much more fluid and indistinct members of an at-risk group. Dealing with an at-risk group led to a considerable increase in the common voice among those facing the therapists: adults or children who shared the same viewpoint.

These two changes pulled the rug out from under any categorical description of the therapeutic interventions. The relationships between the participants and the therapists were unlike those that anthropologists usually describe between Western trauma experts providing aid in non-Western areas (Dwyer and Santikarma, 2007; James, 2004). Rather, the therapeutic interventions turned out to echo the sociopolitical dynamic in Israel. The social position of the National Orthodox Jewish settlers as yeshiva students and the right-wing residents of the Occupied Territories was charged with meaning vis-à-vis the psychologist's social position as a secular, left-wing resident of central Israel. The social workers' position as Bedouin women was charged with meaning vis-à-vis the psychologist's social position as a secular Jewish woman. The bereaved parents' social position as members of the Druze minority was charged with meaning vis-à-vis the secular Judaism of the therapist leading the seminar. The social position of Kibbutz Zikkim's children as part of a communal establishment living near the Gaza Strip was charged with meaning vis-à-vis the therapists living in cities beyond the range of Qassam rocket fire. From these diverse social positions, the participants revealed different subjective experiences, and with them various strategies for understanding, interpreting, and coping with mental vulnerability as a result of prolonged political conflict.

In the next chapter, the clinical definitions of trauma and PTSD are no longer in motion but are rooted in one specific context: the southern town of Sderot.

Chapter Seven

Taking Hold: Resilience Program in the Southern Town of Sderot

They bring their people, get a project for three to four years, accumulate knowledge and experience by working in Sderot and improve their [clinical] tools, and then they present the results of the work they've done here or in any other peripheral location. Moneywise too, this money doesn't stay here; it goes out because outsiders receive these salaries. Other organizations earn this money, and sustain themselves. Then, after three years, what a surprise, instead of being stronger, we are weaker, because the knowledge and money leave. They don't stay here ... the experts leave, the money goes ... we are left depleted, and need to start anew.

> – Nurit Alush, a social worker living in Sderot and daughter of Moroccan immigrants who came to the city in its early years, 7 April 2006

This chapter deals with the most dramatic distance that opened up between the clinical diagnostic concepts of trauma and PTSD and the process of preventing them, through the concepts of "resilience" and "immunization." Alush's remarks indicate how this professional divergence positioned the politics that developed around trauma in Israel within socio-economic and ethnic hierarchies. Alush was addressing the arrival of well-trained senior therapists from ITC and NATAL to assist the local residents with their prolonged exposure to the Qassam rockets. At the same time, she revealed her troublesome feelings in relation to those senior therapists. They indeed wanted to help, she said, but the local distress also served as a platform where they could acquire more experience and enhance their reputations as trauma specialists for the next intervention, next town, next war, and next budget. Nina Gurgi, Alush's friend, continued in the same direction. She voiced how the trauma therapists perceived themselves as being "supermen" who had come to the town to assist "the poor and the ignorant, the quite dumb and scared from Sderot. We have come to save you!"

These arguments by Alush and Gurgi in relation to the trauma aid providers should be understood in a broader historical context. The founding of Sderot in 1953 was part of a nationwide project to establish "development towns," primarily aimed at populating areas near the Israeli borders (Tzfadia and Yiftachel, 2004). Ashkenazi Jews (of European origin), who constituted the dominant group among the state's founders, sent groups of new immigrants to settle these towns, including Sderot. In the first decades, Mizrachim Jews (of Middle Eastern and North African origin, especially from Morocco) were sent to live there. Later, the authorities sent other groups of Jews, those from Ethiopia and the former Soviet Union, particularly from Bukhara and from the Caucasus. As early as the 1950s and 1960s, the welfare discourse referred to the city's population as "disadvantaged" and in need of special resources in order to narrow down the ethnic Ashkenazi-Mizrachi gap. The semantic field used by professionals changed over the years. For example, the reference changed from "distressed youth" to "children at-risk," but the stigma remained the same (Mizrachi, 2004).

The ethnographic tracing of the politics of trauma that developed in Sderot began when this geographic and socio-economic marginality merged with a security issue. Since the onset of the second Palestinian uprising against Israel and its occupation of Palestinian territories in October 2000, thousands of Qassam rockets have been fired from the Palestinian Gaza Strip at the town of Sderot and other settlements in southern Israel. In June 2004, the rockets claimed their first fatalities. A young boy, Afik Ohayon, and his friend's grandfather, Mordechai Yosifov, were killed when a rocket hit the Lilakh preschool in the Neveh Eshkol neighbourhood. Their deaths sparked fear and angry protest in Sderot. The residents protested against the state, claiming its agencies failed to provide them with any protective shield.

A few weeks later, their protest seemed to have borne some fruit. Instead of the Israeli government, the Jewish Federations of North America decided to provide generous funding for trauma therapists from Israeli NGOs, especially NATAL and ITC, to offer mental aid to the local residents. With the financial support of those Jewish Federations, the therapists built a professional program called "community resilience" (*tokhnit hosen kehilati* in Hebrew). In a document distributed to government ministries, the North American Jewish

Federations and municipal offices in southern Israel announced their program as follows:

> In the course of the last four years, the forty thousand residents of Sderot, Sha'ar Hanegev, Hof Ashkelon, Sdot Negev, and Eshkol have become the frontline facing ongoing Palestinian violence. Since the year 2000, over four hundred Qassam rockets have been launched from the Gaza Strip into the area, and many have hit playgrounds, schools, and other population centers. These rockets have not broken the spirit of the residents of Sderot and its neighbouring communities. Despite four years of terror and uncertainty, the grave socioeconomic situation and the high unemployment rate, the city's residents have remained stable and committed to their community ... [The goals of the program are] to build a resilient community and empower Sderot by providing immediate aid in order to manage the intense reactions of the residents to the situation and strengthen their coping skills. (ITC's resilience program, September 2004)

As can be seen, the program was mainly psychological ("managing reactions" and "strengthening coping skills"), and contained at least two paradoxes that aptly expressed the complexity involved in it. First, although the trauma therapists described the residents as desperately in need of help (due to terror, economic problems, and unemployment), they stated that the population's spirit was unbroken. Second, although their goal was to strengthen the community as a whole, they targeted their intervention at individuals. Still, how precisely did they view the designated recipients of their new resilience program? A document published two years later provides clarification:

> We anticipate that at least thirty percent of the city's population was seriously affected by the events and between ten to twenty percent have already suffered long-term and chronic effects of post-trauma symptoms ... In addition to the cases that require direct treatment, we will provide others with psychosocial interventions for the purpose of strengthening their personal and family resilience. (ITC's resilience program, December 2006)

ITC and NATAL, therefore, have drawn a clear connection between the clinical construct of trauma and their intervention in Sderot. They noted a widespread (and differentiated) impact of the rockets on the entire population living next to the Gaza Strip. They based their program on statistics (the percentage of PTSD sufferers), while creating a "victim portfolio" (James, 2004: 132): numerical prediction based on the integration of local characterizations and clinical expertise.

However, at the same time, the professional management of mental vulnerability in Sderot bore a special character. According to the document, the events gravely affected 30 per cent of the city's residents, with 10 to 20 per cent exhibiting long-term symptoms of PTSD. The other 70 per cent, although not showing these symptoms, still presented as requiring professional intervention in order to build up their personal, family, and community "resilience." Thus, the population targeted by these professionals included a minority clinical group that was exhibiting pathological symptoms, as well as a majority group described as preclinical and in need of fortification as a preventive measure. Thus, under these circumstances, a new social expansion of trauma and PTSD was marked. Instead of reactive intervention, the therapists were suggesting proactive intervention. This new strategy for trauma management offered an opportunity to examine an important shift in the politics that had developed around the concept of trauma: from responding to signs of pathology displayed solely by individuals to anticipating clinical symptoms around which pre-emptive actions could be taken in order to immunize an entire town against possible trauma.

In what follows, I examine this transformation from reactive treatment of individuals to building resilience in a community. Which specific communication strategies enabled ITC and NATAL therapists to occupy a new social site for action? How did they convert trauma and PTSD, for the very first time, from a clinical label into a preclinical therapeutic principle? What happened in the course of this process regarding the sociopolitical negotiation between the external therapists and the various groups of residents? How did local caregivers from Sderot and other members from this peripheral community react to the new resilience program offered to them by therapists from Israel's centre?

One Town, Divided Therapeutic Intervention

Since the leaders of the Sderot resilience program (NATAL and ITC) were from neither governmental agencies nor international humanitarian organizations, they allowed themselves to make fine distinctions within the town's population. They split the population into three focal groups, each serving as a new target for therapeutic intervention and a specific kind of treatment. First, the therapists operated a "mobile unit for treatment of traumatized families" throughout the city. Second, they formed "haven rooms" in elementary schools. Third, they ran work-shops for "developing personal resilience" in elementary schools, edu-cation and welfare departments, and in the various neighbourhoods. These interventions corresponded to different levels of proximity to the perceived clinical core of trauma. The levels ranged from the treatment of individuals within families suffering from PTSD to intervention of groups exposed to anxiety experiences preceding PTSD to immuniza-tion of groups against future PTSD.

Moving Aid into the Community:
Mobile Clinic for Treatment of Traumatized Families

From the onset of the resilience program in Sderot, therapists made an effort to identify and treat children and adults exhibiting symptoms of PTSD. However, in January 2007, after several weeks of increasing Qassam rocket fire, these activities took a form that expanded the inter-vention into new realms. At the initiative of the senior clinical psychol-ogist from NATAL, and in cooperation with Sderot's municipal welfare department, a mobile clinic began to operate in the city. Six psycholo-gists (including speakers of Amharic and Russian) travelled in a special van around Sderot once a week, treating families in their homes.

However, this intervention was immediately associated with ethno-class concerns. The experts from NATAL claimed it was a response to the "weaker" groups' tendency to avoid psychotherapeutic ser-vices. The list of families scheduled for the van's visits had been gen-erated from carefully selected applications to the municipal welfare department. Under the trauma therapists' guidance, the department's personnel identified those applications perceived as having at least one member suffering from PTSD.

In operating the mobile unit, the therapists expanded their profes-sional repertoire to include diverse and eclectic therapeutic practices. The therapists conducted an "evaluation of the level of functioning at work, at school, and in emergencies"; taught "skills to contend with and prepare for future stress situations and distress"; identified family members suffering from "very serious distress"; processed individuals' traumatic memories; and showed them how to regulate their feelings and control their physical responses. Besides the specific people in a family that the psychologists targeted for intervention, all members became the focus of intervention and the psychologists offered them a therapeutic "toolkit." Frequently switching between individuals diagnosed with PTSD and the family as a whole, the therapists taught "parenting skills" (keeping a routine and setting rules and boundaries), and sometimes even suggested a "systematic change" in a family's lifestyle.

The therapists' reports revealed the practical applications of their new interventions. The PTSD reports placed clients on an axis of time, spanning past trauma, present consequences, and future outcomes. This enabled the therapists to detail the "main problem," "therapy plan," and "prognosis" for each family. For example, a therapist presented an intervention for a family with three children as follows:

> Main problem: Numerous Qassams hit in the home vicinity. The mother and the two daughters are being treated. The son constantly clings to the mother, is restless, and afraid to be alone even in the bathroom. Therapy plan and prognosis: Work with the son to provide support, and teach him skills to calm down; work with the mother on separation. Medium prognosis. (7 February 2007, Mobile Clinic's Report)

Another report presented a widow and mother of three:

> Main problem: The woman witnessed the hits of several Qassams. Two years ago, her hand was injured, and her granddaughter was killed. Symptoms: Difficulty in sleeping, tension, overexcitement, headaches with no medical finding. Therapy plan and prognosis: Ventilation, ongoing therapeutic and behavioral support in coping with fear; reinforcing strengths and existing support systems. The woman is mature, the prognosis is somewhat poor, but even a partial improvement in her condition is very important. (7 February 2007, Mobile Clinic's Report)

The therapist wrote the following about a divorced mother of five children:

> Main problem: Two months ago a Qassam fell next to the house. Since then the mother has suffered from anxieties and overexcitement most of the time. Once she fainted. She has difficulty sleeping, and blows up at the children for no good reason. Other family members display typical reactions. Therapy plan and prognosis: Work with the mother to give her tools for coping with fear and anxiety, like practising self-defense and logical thinking. Reinforce existing strengths. Good prognosis. (7 February 2007, Mobile Clinic's Report)

This clinical technique demonstrates how the therapists took a very complex, multilayered, sociopolitical experience of violence and suffering and transformed it into emotional symptoms and a treatment plan. Underlying the clinical symptoms such as anxiety, physical clinging, overexcitement, and anger, damaged property, broken glass, blasts, actual injury, and loss of life due to the Qassam rocket fire were downplayed as therapists transferred them from the political to the new clinical arena. Thus, the mobile clinic marked the beginning of treating trauma as a new type of medical condition; not only did the therapists isolate the mental problems of families and of individuals within families (Bracken, 1998; Kleinman, 1995; Young, 1995), they also helped to expand the mode of intervention. Instead of patients coming to a clinic, the therapists travelled around via a mobile clinic. The chosen title of "mobile clinic" testifies to the emphasis on portability and reflects an effort to acquire legitimacy similar to that of emergency vehicles.

Intervention at the Onset of Trauma: "Haven Rooms"

Designing haven rooms in elementary schools, the second practice applied under the resilience program, conveyed an effort to intervene at an early stage of trauma. The purpose of these rooms was to provide tranquility to offset the emergence of anxiety that was a characteristic of this early stage. Each school was asked to allocate a room (usually a storeroom or a counsellor's office) that could be redesigned according to the therapists' guidelines. With the investment of a few thousand dollars each, schools emptied the rooms of their contents and filled them with a pale-hued carpet and large, colourful pillows for seating. In addition, therapists placed dolls in various nooks and scattered around selected books and games that might enable the children to reference feelings, such as fear, sorrow, anger, and happiness.

The schools' pedadogic counsellors planned to conduct various activities in these rooms. These activities included occasional talks with the schools' counsellors at anxious moments following a Qassam attack, a series of preplanned talks, movement therapy, and group discussions (insofar as participants were capable) about emotional distress. The director of the project, Meir Shapiro, an educational psychologist supported by the American Jewish Distribution Committee (JDC), explained:

The program was built in order to respond to the emotional situation, particularly among children from elementary schools ... When we got to the schools, we understood that the situation was extremely serious. There was an increase in violence, tension, and anxiety. It was something much broader, and more damaging to everything, to everyone. So we expanded our activity and said that we would carry out intervention with all sorts of children in whom we see and feel the effect ... [This means] that the children are not referred to therapy, but the therapy is brought into the schools. (Interview, 20 June 2006)

In describing the rationale for the establishment of the haven rooms, the expansion of the trauma treatment was evident. The goal of the therapy program was to bring the clinic to the school and to the community itself. The intervention, organized as a part of collaboration between ITC and JDC, treated trauma as an overall condition of social reality throughout Israel:

In the existing situation in Israel, many children and adolescents are exposed to traumatic events as a result of Qassam rockets and continued acts of terror. The haven rooms program in the schools is intended to improve the coping and competence of students, parents and teachers in ongoing traumatic and emergency situations ... The overall goal is to create an optimal physical environment in the schools ... The haven room has added value as it is a concrete physical place that serves as an emotional "safety room" for the students. (Haven Rooms Foundation Document, 2006)

The new room was a distinct space in each school, permanently marked and designed to achieve an emotional objective: tranquility. As such, this new strategy of intervention blurred the pathological symptoms upon which the intervention was founded: the numerous expressions of distress that the therapists had identified in schools ("increase in violence, tension, and anxiety") led them to the conclusion that Qassam rocket fire was hurting "everyone." Similar to the mobile units, the emotional semantics around the haven rooms echoed the "security" discourse in Israel. The haven rooms drew their legitimacy from the widespread safety shelters that had been constructed within homes and public buildings all over Israel for many years. Furthermore, using security-related concepts to describe the rooms softened any stigma people might have associated with entering them. The rooms became an integral part of schools, so the temporary labelling of being "under treatment" dissipated when the children returned to their classrooms and the routine of their studies.

Immunizing the Town: Workshops for "Developing Resilience"

The most innovative therapeutic practice implemented in Sderot was the workshops for developing personal and community resilience. The aim of these workshops was to prevent acute trauma prior to its onset. Yoni Forman, a psychologist who led a workshop for the principal and ten teachers at Hatorah Elementary School, articulated the rationale:

> We are in a very complex and demanding period with the entire nation in prolonged trauma for several years. Those at risk are our children, who don't always understand who's fighting whom, and who can't always bear the threat to their and their parents' lives. We believe in working and strengthening the teaching staff, not because they need reinforcement, but in order to remind them of a few things, to give them a tool or two so they can do some work prior to and after [attacks]. Also, the more we invest in advance, the better people will be immunized, medically and emotionally, and the better they will hold up, and the less injured and upset they will become. (10 August 2005, Field Notes)

Forman constructed the reality that the residents of Sderot were facing as part of the larger reality of the trauma that the entire nation was experiencing. Next, he identified the most vulnerable group prone to acute trauma – children. Forman argued that the children lacked an understanding of the situation and were in need of better coping skills. The paradoxical combination of both strength and weakness, as noted earlier in this chapter, was prominent here as well. Forman, the psychologist, claimed that teachers needed minimal intervention in order to help the children, and that this would guarantee significant results. Furthermore, similar to the analogy between mobile clinics and emergency vehicles, and between haven rooms and group safety shelters, the analogy between mental resilience and medical immunization served as an important strategy for Forman and other professionals to persuade people of the necessity of this new therapeutic intervention.

Forman and his team from NATAL created a booklet to guide the psychologists in their intervention work. The booklet clarified that the intervention workshops would be a series of exercises aimed at building up resilience to potential distress. The techniques focused on developing various dimensions of self-control, specifically regarding emotional, cognitive, and behavioural management (Gaines, 1992). On the emotional level, the goal was to "enrich our emotional vocabulary, sharpen the distinction between different emotions, and make speaking about feelings acceptable." The therapists taught special techniques directed at managing fear and anger. Against fear, the booklet instructed the participants to imagine a "safe place" where they would feel "protected and loved." Further, it explained that anger was not isolated from accompanying thoughts like "I was treated unfairly or unjustly," and that it was liable to be expressed in aggressive behaviour, or as an emotion that "began with a drizzle and became a flood." The participants learned how to "acquire self-control, and direct anger into positive channels." On the cognitive level, participants learned definitions of "stress"; used scales (numbers and colours) to express stress; developed coping strategies (organizing thoughts and collecting information); used religious faith to give meaning to events; and employed positive thinking to strengthen optimism and competence. On the behavioural level, participants practised relaxation, guided imagery, and strengthening social ties for the purpose of "building social resilience."

Ethnic and Political Negotiations

In order to understand the negotiations that developed around the resilience program in Sderot, it is important to consider how the lead senior psychologists portrayed their interventions. For example, Eli Magid, one of the senior psychologists who was involved in the program from the outset, gave the following report to his colleagues at their annual meeting:

> In Sderot, we have gradually become the representatives of mental health. We operate twenty-one projects there. We are involved in all the schools, with a budget of 750,000 [Israeli shekels]. Three thousand students go through the program we have developed. This is our direction for the future, not individual work, but reaching large groups by means of professional work in the community. (NATAL, 29 September 2005, Field Notes)

Magid expressed the crucial change with the use of the clinical concepts of trauma and PTSD, "not individual work, but reaching large groups," as a great success. However, transforming these clinical concepts from the private sphere into the community sphere triggered intensive debate and resistance, especially on the part of local caregivers and residents.

Local Caregivers Explain: "From the start they built a certain type of ghetto here"

A tense dynamic developed between the visiting members from ITC and NATAL and the local caregivers, some of whom had worked in Sderot for many years. On the one hand, the external therapists, clinical psychologists, and psychiatrists belonging to the NGOs of central Israel were in a senior position and of higher professional status in comparison to the status of the local caregivers work in Sderot. The local caregivers were mostly social workers and school counsellors. Moreover, funded by North American federations, the external experts had access to financial and organizational resources, which turned them into attractive partners for collaboration, especially in the relatively poor socio-economic context of Israel's southern periphery. On the other hand, since the local caregivers held key positions in the town, the external experts considered them as key figures for implementing the resilience program. Nonetheless, despite their lower professional status, or perhaps precisely because of that, the local caregivers refused to be passive assistants of the program and continuously debated its relevancy and effectiveness.

Anastasia Kima, for example, a psychiatrist who immigrated to Israel from the former Soviet Union and was serving as director of the mental health clinic in Sderot, described the local population:

> Sderot's population is problematic and complex, even without the Qassams. The Qassams intensify the very difficult things that are specific to the place. Immigrants, without going into detail ... the least successful type of immigrants, and of course unemployment, a lower cultural level, a population that is behaviourally problematic, alcoholism, drugs, children of a lesser God – these are the Sderot people ... to a high percentage, I believe. If you add to this the impact of the Qassams or anything else, you get the answer ... I believe that from the start they built a sort of a ghetto for a certain kind of people here. They forgot to mix them with better material, and this is the result. (Interview, 26 June 2006)

According to Kima, the trauma resulting from the rocket attacks was merely an addition to the many other serious problems the Sderot people were facing. She did not use abstract, politically correct language for socio-economic indicators, but referred to the local population with a series of social-ethnic labels, such as "unemployment," "lower cultural level," and "a population that is behaviourally problematic."

The director of the municipal psychological services, Reut Armon, an Israeli-born educational psychologist who had worked in Sderot for a long time, was also inclined to view the trauma symptoms as an addition to a series of existing problems. However, she used different explanations for distress:

> The community of Sderot is insufficiently strong on many levels. There are difficult groups here ... new immigrants, very serious welfare cases, impoverished groups, many single-parent families, many families receiving help from the welfare department and mental health authorities. These people have been shattered by situations of emergency and crisis ... They have no inner strength to cope ... Now, when a mother reacts badly, automatically her six or seven children collapse with her! It's simple – I see this in lots of families – when the mother cries all the time, doesn't function, is stressed and begins screaming when she hears the siren, her children cling to her anxiously. She is unable to contain herself and her children fall apart with her too. How we are to help on this level is a really big problem. In addition, we don't have Russian-speaking staff, and there are Ethiopians too. It is a population that isn't used to getting such help. They aren't psychologically minded, [they are not] people who know how to receive help. (Interview, 11 June 2006)

Unlike Kima, the psychiatrist and director of mental health, Armon did not refer to the residents as problematic "material" but as individuals lacking the "inner strength to cope." She also argued that the residents were unreachable given the lack of therapists who could speak their languages and because they had the wrong mindset regarding therapeutic interventions as "they aren't psychologically minded." Furthermore, she explained that children suffered a breakdown together with their mothers since they followed their mothers' anxious reactions. Once again, though for different reasons, Armon depicted the resilience program as ineffective for the local residents.

These diverse views about the appropriate treatment for the suffering population – among the local professionals, between them and the external professionals – were part of the politics evolving around the new intervention plan. In particular, the local professionals argued that organizational interests inappropriately determined the latest new applications of PTSD (see James 2004, on Haiti). For example, Sharon

Keinan, born in an agricultural settlement (a *moshav*) near Sderot and working as an educational psychologist at the local infant welfare clinic, said:

> There are all sorts of power games and contests between organizations and all sorts of things that ultimately made us feel that we were left alone in the struggle ... In the end, when there is a need, we are there and that's it. Only we are there. It is true that they came with good intentions and with money, but for them alone ... In no way did this [intervention] empower the caregivers here, who, unfortunately, have become the real experts in PTSD. (Interview, 4 July 2006)

Shira Saban, a social worker in the municipal welfare department who was born in Sderot, underscored the financial issues and the misfit nature of the program in harsher terms:

> Most people who came to Sderot in the beginning, came to cash in, so they could make money ... Lots came, many organizations. There was extraordinary disorder ... It was a mess ... They decided that this was needed, but this is not the true need of Sderot ... They came with their experience; the experience is excellent, but it's not necessarily right for Sderot. (Interview, 18 July 2006)

In contrast to the external therapists' universal and neutral-scientific language (e.g., in their founding documents), Saban pointed to the intervention's political context, to issues of professional prestige, and to the economic interests of the therapists and the NGOs alike.

Critical Residents: "It suits Ashkenazim, this music"

The debate over the nature of the psychological aid offered to the residents of Sderot was also expressed during the interventions themselves. In a workshop for school counsellors working in Sderot's elementary schools, two external psychologists tried to explain how to prevent anger among children following Qassam rocket attacks. However, the local counsellors objected:

> BEN EFRON (PSYCHOLOGIST): There are many obstacles from the outside, but take responsibility for your position ... You should believe in yourselves, and that's a matter of choice. It's not all external forces.

OREN KAPLAN (PSYCHOLOGIST): When there is a serious emergency, when there is great distress, people think there is only one possible reaction. However, in emergencies there are all sorts of options. I can influence my feelings through thoughts ... influencing instead of being influenced.

SIGAL AMIR (LOCAL COUNSELLOR): [But] anger, for example, is not a bad thing. It's a sign that something needs to be changed. (Other counsellors to her left and right nod in agreement, and cry out "right, right") (20 February 2006, Field Notes)

Whereas the psychologists tried to teach inner control of emotions and, as they later explained, not to allow anger to influence the residents' behaviour, the local counsellors tried to underscore how the expression of anger was good, serving as a potential generator of change.

Encounters between the therapists and the residents further emphasized the class and ethnic differences between local and external professionals. As it turned out, the residents constantly challenged the resilience rationale and rejected a multitude of intervention strategies: the invitation "to imagine a safe place," the use of "emotional security shelters," the demand to "give a positive interpretation to the experience," and the suggestion to "direct anger into positive channels." One example occurred during a workshop for nursing caregivers in November 2006 one day after a rocket hit Sderot, killing a resident and seriously injuring a security officer who lost his leg. Michael Shonfeld, a psychologist, started talking about belief and commitment as ways to cope with the situation. The participants found it hard to listen, talking instead about the broader politics involved in living in this troubled peripheral city:

MICHAEL SHONFELD (PSYCHOLOGIST): It's important to teach values: "Why do we stay here? Why don't we move?"

BAT-SHEVA MIZRACHI (in a loud voice, agitated): What do you think, that everyone can get up and leave? Where to? Try selling a house in Sderot nowadays. People have no choice!

GEULA SHIRAZI (ANOTHER PARTICIPANT): Not everybody stays because of ideology, saying, "We'll stay and fight!"... In the south we are the state's forsaken children. (November 2006, Field Notes)

When the psychologist suggests relying upon "values" in order to strengthen resilience, the residents immediately replied by pointing to the economic constraints that forced people to stay. In a workshop for the Neveh Eshkol neighbourhood where the first fatalities from Qassam rockets occurred, psychologist Yoseph Varburg asked about inner versus outer strategies of coping. Residents replied with political protest, emphasizing ethnic differences between themselves and the external therapists:

YOSEPH VARBURG (PSYCHOLOGIST): Who is responsible for calming us
– the government or ourselves?

SALVA ZUBAKOV (A RUSSIAN IMMIGRANT WHO ARRIVED IN
SDEROT A FEW YEARS BEFORE THE PALESTINIAN ROCKETS
BEGAN; angrily): The government! Not us ... The Qassams make the
population [miserable] – They don't believe in the government. I will try
not to send my son and daughter to the army. I have no faith ... Our plan
is to learn English and leave Israel ... What do they say in the centre of
the country? "Ah, there are Qassams over there." As if we are second-
class citizens.

YOSEPH VARBURG (smiling): There's a lot of anger today!

DEVORAH FISHBAIN (AN ISRAELI-BORN, LONG-STANDING
RESIDENT): I feel that all the governments – they want ... the population
to be helpless ... Perhaps we need to set up our Sderot squads, and start
firing Qassams too.

SALVA ZUBAKOV: Yesterday they said, "You are Sderot, you are good."
Today they say, "You are Sderot, you are garbage." How can I send my
son to the army? ... Who will thank you if you have no son because he
served in the army? Who? You will be invited to Jerusalem on Memorial
Day to stand in the background.

RIVKA TAGANIA (AN ETHIOPIAN IMMIGRANT WHO ARRIVED IN
SDEROT IN THE EARLY 1980S): Everybody says about us in Sderot,
"A few Moroccans, a few Ethiopians, and a few Israelis who didn't know
what they were doing."

YOSEPH VARBURG: I planned to give you some practical tools, to help
people calm down if you see they are stressed. I want to put on some
soft, pleasant music and each will do what he or she wants.

RIVKA TAGANIA (sarcastically): It suits Ashkenazim [European Jews],
this music. (4 July 2006, Field Notes)

In this dialogue, the tension between the psychologist's intention to build resilience and the participants' political standpoint was clear (see Han, 2004; Zarowsky, 2004). In contrast to the former's efforts to reshape the subjective reality of the residents, the latter pointed out the difficulties of the external environment. While the nursing caregivers cited economic weakness as the reason for staying, residents expressed even stronger alienation through explicit political protest against the government, the army, and other symbols of the state. Devorah suggested taking violent measures; and Salva said he would try to keep his children away from compulsory military service and told the group that his family's survival depended on learning English, so they could leave Israel. Ethnic expressions also articulated these oppositions. The primary example was Rivka's argument according to the therapeutic tool of calming music suited for Ashkenazim (European Jews), not the Mizrachim (Middle Eastern and North African Jews) of Sderot.

Conclusion

The professional effort to build resilience among the residents of Sderot moved away from the clinical nucleus of trauma, as it happened earlier under terms such as secondary trauma (discussed in chapter 5) and at-risk groups (discussed in chapter 6). However, in Sderot the experts sought to "purchase a grip," both literally and figuratively. Thanks to broad philanthropic funding, the NGOs established long-term and comprehensive aid interventions in the community. Accordingly, the therapeutic target of the resilience program was not the individual suffering from PTSD who was treated at a clinic (such as the IDF's soldiers from chapter 4), nor a specific group assigned a distinct social status (such as the bereaved parents from chapter 6), but rather an entire urban community. Thus, the resilience interventions among the residents of Sderot embodied another turning point in the globalization of PTSD (Breslau, 2004; Fassin and Rechtman, 2009) and in the local politics surrounding it. In one way or another, all the residents of Sderot became the target of therapeutic intervention. The experts directed the program not only towards the "clinical minority," those who had already developed symptoms related to PTSD, but also towards the "pre-clinical majority." The pre-clinical majority were those individuals who were still quite far from being diagnosed with PTSD but who the therapists thought would benefit from a proactive prevention program focused on "building resilience" and "social immunization." These new therapeutic practices marked a transition from the post-traumatic to the pre-traumatic, and from treating suffering individuals to strengthening – and immunizing – a community.

As they did with PTSD, Israeli trauma experts brought the concept of resilience with them from North America (Egeland, Carlson, and Sroufe, 1993; Kobasa, 1982; Richardson, 2002). If trauma is defined as "the great psychiatric narrative of our era" (Luhrmann, 2010: 722), this idea of developing coping skills in the face of adversity is its most persuasive counter-narrative. The clinical construct of resilience represented a shift from dealing with risk factors and psychopathology to focusing on skills of adaptation, identifying strengths, and developing internal and external resources. However, as a result of the ongoing Arab–Israeli conflict, the resilience program in Sderot carried with it national significance. From the rhetoric they used, it seemed clear that the experts understood that resilience was not only a psychological issue but also an expression of the local ethos in the form of "national morale" and "patriotism" (see Ya'ar and Peleg, 2007).

Framed within the idea of resilience, new therapeutic language conveyed this expanded version of trauma and PTSD along with prevention strategies. To the strictly psychiatric symptoms of PTSD, experts added diverse indicators from the related fields of health and education, such as "harsh reactions." In response to this generalized "trauma," they formulated various therapeutic terms, including "psycho-social assistance," "calming down," and "strengthening personal and family resilience." In addition, the well-known Israeli security discourse provided the anchor and justification for the intervention analogies. For instance, mobile units and haven rooms resonate with emergency vehicles and safety rooms, and, in Hebrew, the mental *hosen* (resilience) closely resembles the biomedical *hisun* (immunization). Even more importantly, attaching resilience to PTSD replicates cultural debate over contradictory depictions of the Jewish-Israeli national ethos. Whereas PTSD fits the victimization of the collective, rooted in the Holocaust of European Jewry, resilience fits the Zionist idea of the "new Jew," which challenges the presumed passivity of exiled Jews (Kidron, 2004).

The program in Sderot achieved this new clinical-social, national-therapeutic target by dividing the aid program into three forms of interventions: mobile units coming to homes, haven rooms being placed in schools, and workshops for developing resilience techniques being offered to diverse groups of residents. Each of these interventions provided a different medicalization process of the local distress and, at the same time, embodied some sociocultural content. The activity of the mobile clinic gave rise to the classic medicalization process as usually described in anthropological research (Bracken, 1998; Kleinman,

1995; Pupavac, 2001; Young, 1995). The shattered glass, blast injuries, and loss of life experienced by the mobile clinic's patients, due to the violent political conflict between Palestinians and Jews, translated into a series of mental symptoms (anxiety, hyper-arousal, and outbursts of rage). However, this medicalization process did not play out at a clinic as usual but rather inside the home, moving from the level of the individual to the level of the entire family.

Similarly, the establishment of haven rooms in the schools gave rise to a medicalization process, but this time of the space. A specific place in the school was marked and defined as devoted to achieving an emotional goal: tranquility. Through this positive term, "haven room" blurred the negative justification for its establishment, which was the severe distress among the children. Consequently, the room enabled a "temporary medicalization." The room marked the children for only the short period while they were in it, and then that association dissolved when they returned to class.

The third and last process of medicalization occurred during the workshops for developing personal resilience. Through psychosocial activities, the therapists carried out medicalization without pathology, marking without a marker. Pursuant to a general professional concern regarding the future development of PTSD symptoms from rocket fire, the program exposed many schoolchildren, local caregivers, and diverse groups of residents to a complex educational process of acquiring and practising emotional, cognitive, and behavioural skills.

The diffusion of this new coupling – resilience versus trauma – into daily life through these three practices of intervention seemed to be a local manifestation of what Venesa Pupavac calls "therapeutic governance" (2001). Several NGOs and philanthropic agencies marshalled their resources for the sake of trauma management in one local town. They created several channels of assistance, directed towards the town's residents regardless of diagnostic clinical symptoms. A blurring of the lines between the clinical signs of trauma and PTSD and a series of social signs (such as socio-economic status and ethnicity) helped the therapists stabilize emotional processes on a large scale. This blurring contributed indirectly to the social well-being in the town, despite the ongoing threat of the Qassam rockets.

However, two qualities of the aid program in Sderot weakened this categorical analysis. First, the new diffusion of trauma, PTSD, and resilience in the town was articulated from the "bottom up" because a central guiding hand did not coordinate it. The various NGOs established their projects independently of each other with hardly any organized collaboration. For example, separate organizations operated the haven rooms and resilience workshops. Still, shared dialogues between the local and external professionals made these projects possible, and all the projects functioned in the context of therapeutic, geopolitical, and ethnic power struggles.

Second, despite the apparent cooperation among the various players, who all belonged to the same national framework, they redefined their competing social identities through the negotiations around the new resilience program. The professional hierarchy between the local and external professionals resonated with the Israeli geopolitical and ethno-national hierarchies (see Tzfadia and Yiftachel, 2004). The Sderot residents perceived the external experts as biased on many accounts. They believed the external professional represented the centre instead of the periphery, they were linked to the upper-middle instead of the lower-middle class or even a lower socio-economic status, and they were predominantly of Ashkenazi origin instead of North African, Russian, or Ethiopian origin. Thus, in this case, the external experts were not the exclusive brokers of trauma (James, 2004). Instead, the local professionals constantly questioned, mediated, and negotiated with the therapists regarding their position as gatekeepers for receiving aid. Directors of Sderot's mental health clinics, educational psychologists, welfare department social workers, and school educational counsellors did not readily accept the new PTSD diagnosis and the new resilience program for the residents they served. They pointed to the financial, professional, and political motivations of the external professionals. In addition, they defended the alternative diagnoses and interventions they had been using for years, such as "a difficult population" and "not psychologically minded" to underscore the local population's social marginality and economic difficulties.

Moreover, the Sderot residents placed their suffering in the context of their peripheral status in Israeli society. They protested against the inappropriate place to which they had been assigned in the national narrative of Israel. They expressed their bitter resentment of the gap between the rhetoric of the state agencies that referred to them as pioneers living on Israel's southern periphery, on the front line of the violent conflict with militant Palestinian organizations, and their marginal socioeconomic and ethnic position in Israeli society. Thus, like Ethiopian refugees in Somalia, they associated their suffering with issues of social injustice (Zarowsky, 2004) and objected to the individualization, psychologization, and depoliticization of their problems, as entailed by the new trauma, PTSD, and resilience interventions. They preferred protection by means of solidarity and the local assistance that emerged within the town. Furthermore, they demanded a change in more than their inner mental reality. They opted to politicize emotions, such as anger, and to mobilize political action that the external professionals tried to thwart. Still, although the residents challenged the therapeutic interventions, their protest differed from other cases reported in anthropological literature. In other instances, residents opposed the correlation drawn by professionals between PTSD diagnosis and those who were entitled to relief (Dwyer and Santikarma, 2007; James, 2004). In Sderot, by contrast, everyone was entitled and invited to receive aid. The only distinction was that the therapists distinguished between types of aid, not between those who were and were not entitled to get help. Accordingly, the Sderot residents protested against the new expanded version of trauma and PTSD and the ambitious resilience program associated with it.

Chapter Eight

A Nation on the Couch:
Treading Cautiously around
Sensitive Clinical and Political Domains

In the summer of 2014, another violent eruption occurred between Israel and the Palestinian military organization of Hamas. Under the title "Protective Edge," the IDF launched a military operation in the Gaza Strip in response to Hamas rocket fire and the threat of underground tunnels. During those tragic days, one phenomenon attracted my attention as an anthropologist. Dozens of hotlines suddenly appeared, with phone numbers and details of aid services published during the endless hours of Israeli news: Consultation Center for Anxiety by Clalit Health Services, Emotional Support Hotline for Parents in Distress, Consulting for Parents of Preschool Children by Women's International Zionist Organization. These and other hotlines invited adults, the elderly, children, and the general public to pick up the phone and, free of charge, share their emotional experiences of being under constant sirens and rocket fire with mental health experts. Alongside the growing public awareness of the mental condition of trauma, the appearance of all of these hotlines is the ultimate illustration of the critical shift in the professional approach towards mental vulnerability under Israel's current security circumstances.

The journey described throughout the chapters of this book was born out of the attempt to look behind the scenes of this change, deep into the politics and pragmatics that evolved around the new diffusion of trauma and PTSD into the daily life in Israel. By using anthropological tools such as participant observations, in-depth interviews, and text analysis, I tried to shed light on those moments when clinical concerns interwove with changing social circumstances, to examine the specific social relations that developed between various social players, and to look at the ways of communication that evolved from these moments of intersection.

The first part of the book addressed the political dimension of the professional management of security-based trauma in Israel through an in-depth description of the establishment of two new aid agencies, both of which were NGOs. The need to adapt the clinical concept of trauma to the changing circumstances of the Arab–Israeli conflict and to adjust to the challenging economic conditions of being dependent on donations for survival (Shamir, 2008; Silber, 2008) led to ongoing negotiations among the trauma experts (chapter 1) and between them and other social players, such as state agencies (also chapter 1), donors (chapter 2), and marketing advisers (chapter 3). All of those social players have become "competing partners" in the negotiations over the meaning of security-based trauma and over the allocation of financial and organizational resources. Within this new framework of tense dialogues, trauma has turned into a fluid category, moving back and forth between two poles of meanings. One pole was the narrow, universal meaning of psychiatric diagnosis that applied to a minority. The second was the perception of trauma as a communal experience tied to a specific place, culture, and nation and thus relevant to the vast majority.

The second part of the book focused on the pragmatic dimension of the professional management of trauma, while tracing several different intervention strategies. I showed how, out of the new organizational agencies, the first strategy addressed the primary context in which trauma awareness emerged in Israeli society: the IDF (see Bilu and Witztum, 2000; Solomon, 1993). By means of incremental steps of treating, documenting, researching, and identifying, the therapists sought to fight their way to what had become a fortified citadel: the mental symptoms of combat soldiers, old and young. As such, they made trauma accessible as a concept to various target audiences of soldiers, a concept that could help them contend with the moral and social questions that military service posed (chapter 4).

From this first divergence, additional strategies for dealing with security-based mental vulnerability were designed. These strategies extended further and further away from the clinical home base, namely, the DSM as the canonical text of Western psychiatry and the clinic as the classic setting for therapeutic intervention. Through softer and more flexible definitions of trauma than the iconic one of PTSD – such as secondary trauma (chapter 5), at-risk groups (chapter 6), and resilience and "immunization" (chapter 7) – the experts and therapists from NATAL and ITC expanded their scope and range of professional activity. Based on semi-clinical definitions, they implemented practices of diagnosis, treatment, and prevention without any necessary connection to the existence of clinical symptoms.

Thus, under the intense sociopolitical reality of Israel, the whole "range from the intimate sphere of family systems to the wider arenas of neighborhood, community, [and the] nation" (Kirmayer, 2015: 388) was demonstrated within one national context. This multi-sited ethnography has made it clear how far the professional approach to trauma has shifted from strict, diagnostic categories that could only be applied in a limited way – that is, based on hard evidence. Rather, a metamorphosis in the professional therapy of trauma has occurred based on three main components. First, a network has developed around the mental condition of trauma. This network is comprised of mental health experts, state agencies, municipal leaders, donors, and a marketing team. Second, the strict psychiatric label, previously relevant only to those diagnosed with the disorder, has broadened into a new social category. This new category is infused with cultural and historical elements, and thus is relevant to the majority of Israelis. Third, the professional scope of activity has extended from interventions aimed at particular individuals to include entire communities and even the nation, far beyond its original clinical basis. Above all, the new diffusion of trauma and PTSD into Israel's daily life represents a story of a medical mission, fuelled and shaped by a powerful national narrative that, in its fulfilment, is repeatedly challenged by the social, cultural, and religious divides of Israeli society.

The aim of this eighth and concluding chapter is to examine this metamorphosis of trauma in light of the two bodies of literature addressing the globalization of trauma. Similar to other national settings around the globe, trauma management in Israel has revealed the inevitable connection between treating mental vulnerability and dealing anew with the ever-present moral and economic dynamics. Nevertheless, it seems that Israel has challenged both anthropological accounts in regard to providing aid across social boundaries.

The first anthropological body of literature emphasizes trauma management in relation to humanitarian discourse and to international relations between Western and non-Western countries (Breslau, 2004; Fassin and Rechtman, 2009; James, 2004). In contrast to this account, I have demonstrated how trauma has been tied to the power struggle within a single national context. Israel's unique demographic structure and ethno-national stratification has created well-established and bitter rifts (see Shafir and Peled, 2002). The processes of diagnosis, treatment, and prevention of traumatic symptoms, as well as decisions regarding the meaning of trauma and allocation of resources, rested upon these internal rifts. This dynamic has given the professional management of trauma in Israel its own particular features and outcomes.

The second anthropological body of literature emphasizes how trauma has become a new marker of national identity. However, this seems to be ineffective at characterizing Israel's use of this clinical term. This marker of national identity was effective regarding the extensive trauma management in the U.S. following the September 11 attacks (Alexander, 2004; Young, 2007) and the South African conceptual use of trauma within the framework of the reconciliation process (Wilson, 2000). Conversely, Israeli trauma management took place with regard to both a violent *and* prolonged political conflict. In this environment, trauma management required another method to maintain the national narrative of Israel as a Jewish state. From the start, the moral engine the experts at NATAL and ITC applied situated trauma inside the basic Zionist ethos of "we the Jews" versus "them the Arabs." Therefore, doubts and dilemmas cropped up in connection with providing mental aid to the Palestinian citizens of Israel as in the case of the Second Lebanon War (chapter 1). However, it has also become clear that experiencing trauma as a result of being exposed to the same violent attacks as the Jews serves as a new means for Arab minorities in Israel to take a more active role in the national narrative of Israel. Furthermore, even within the boundaries of the Jewish-Israeli community, the use of trauma intersected with the social class and ethno-national hierarchies in Israel. It turned out that veiled messages also accompanied the unifying message of trauma management in Israel. These messages reflected the existence of power struggles between "Ashkenazim" and "Mizrachim," secular and religious, and men and women.

Thus, the particular features and consequences of the political and pragmatic dimensions that evolved around security-based trauma and PTSD in Israel seemed to invite a more nuanced interpretation of the local use of these clinical definitions, one that is sensitive to the various local micro levels in which trauma therapy has been applied within a single national site. In addition, it must take into account the diverse practices that experts and therapists employ within those specific sites. In what follows, I try to offer an interpretation of this kind by exposing the two local system of meanings between which the current professional management of trauma became situated – the individualistic and the collectivistic. As the new diffusion of trauma has the ability to contain both of these, I examine how this process has led to a new "therapeutic contract" between aid providers and aid receivers.

Between Individualism and Collectivism: Orchestrating a New Therapeutic Contract

The critical shift in the professional therapy of trauma in Israel should be viewed as being embedded within the intersection between two different belief systems: individualism versus collectivism. The former belief system emphasizes the autonomy of the individual as an independent player, while the latter emphasizes the group or the community as the most meaningful framework within which the individual exists. Both of these belief systems have strongly shaped daily life in Israel, and each one of them has been strongly influenced by particular historical, ethnic, and sociocultural forces associated with Israeli society.

Understandably, dealing with trauma under the current security circumstances of Israel echoes the individualistic world view. This liberal-oriented emphasis on the individual as the main object of analysis first began to emerge in Israel after the harsh outcomes of the 1973 War. A new legitimacy for local NGOs to promote human rights discourse emerged at that time (Bilu and Witztum, 2000; Kimmerling, 1993). Local activists in Israel, like their colleagues around the globe, tried to break through the collective boundaries of social identity and morality. Their goal was to take action against the very well-known division in Israel of "we the Jews" versus "them the Arabs." Furthermore, the globalization of recent decades has given the individualistic world view and its local advocates a strong tailwind. Sociologists and anthropologists have often indicated that "a sense of boundarylessness" (Beck, 2006: 3) or a process of "de-territorialization" characterize the social world in the late twentieth century (Appadurai, 1996: 52). They argue that these processes have turned the nation-state into an entity with ever-decreasing power in the lives of individuals and groups. With this claim, they have provided additional justification for the strength of the individualistic orientation as an organizing framework for contemporary social life. Within it, the individual's rights and duties, along with his or her position in the social world, are no longer directly or necessarily come from his or her sense of group belonging, such as to a nation, ethnicity, or class. Instead, each individual is a product of being an autonomous subject, with a relatively high degree of freedom to make his or her decisions and choices.

The intersection between the therapeutic language and the individualistic world view have long been familiar to social scientists. For example, in her book *Saving the Modern Soul: Therapy, Emotions, and the Culture of Self-Help* (2008), Eva Illouz points to the success of psychology in penetrating the core institutions of American society: the state, the corporation, the media, and the family. Illouz explains this process as due to the capacity of the therapeutic discourse to offer not only an interpretative framework but also practical tools for managing the difficulties that have arisen from the individualistic spirit in general, and from norms that characterize the modern lifestyle in particular. The array of choices and conflicting expectations that the individual faces make the therapeutic language an anchor for many people. Illouz describes how the development of various emotional skills has turned into a new resource for obtaining social and material rewards within the family or labour market, and from that achieving a sense of self-fulfilment and well-being.

In the wake of the broad cultural analysis offered by Illouz (2008), it is evident that the professional contention with trauma under the current security circumstances of Israel bears a clear individual cast. Being rooted in scientific knowledge perceived as objective and neutral (see Young, 1995; Kleinman, 1995), the professional management of trauma provided a crucial recognition and a distinctive place to the individual. The ethnographic descriptions offered throughout the chapters of this book have exposed the unique power of this individual-therapeutic course of action, not within the family or labour market (Illouz, 2008) but in the context of a violent and prolonged political conflict. By its very nature, such a conflict tends to highlight attributes of group identity according to place, history, culture, and tradition, and to deepen senses of national belonging. In this highly politicized situation, the diagnostic categories of trauma and PTSD provided social acknowledgement and aid resources only on behalf of the existence of mental vulnerability and distress. After all, among the critical theories in the social sciences, this was the very fundamental argument against the therapeutic discourse. Anthropologists and sociologists have claimed that under "pathological labelling," such as trauma and PTSD, the mental health discourse has created a process of de-contextualization: isolating the individual from any broader social context, distancing him or her from any moral or historical background, and marking him or her as a potential carrier of disorder (Bracken, 1998; Kleinman, 1995; Pupavac, 2001).

However, in the exceptional circumstances of the Israeli context, the implementation of clinical concepts takes a more complex and ambiguous meaning. The strength of trauma and PTSD as narrow psychiatric labels has turned them into effective means of getting away from the political and the controversial in an environment specfically full of politics and controversy. Thus, it seems that in Israel, a new political meaning was given to psychiatric labels as their implementation allowed creating a kind of common denominator among different populations in the country. The National Orthodox Jew who was forcibly evacuated from his or her home during the Disengagement Plan; the Bedouin social worker endangered by Qassam rockets; the grief-stricken Druze father mourning his son's death; the resident of Sderot threatened by Qassam rockets; the Palestinian resident exposed to Katyusha rockets; and the combat soldier who had been captured or was coping with losing a comrade – all of them have been recognized, all of them have been labelled. In this sense, the clinical concepts of trauma and PTSD became a new accepted coding for various forms of political suffering to be marked and therefore emphasized the common humanity of different ethnic populations, while overcoming long and deep divisions of "us" versus "them."

Alongside this creative association of trauma and PTSD with individualistic orientation is the local application of these terms that resonate with the collectivistic orientation. Contrary to the individualistic world view, this framework is strongly rooted within the narrow boundaries of a particular ethno-national group. Even during the last few decades and despite the powerful processes of globalization, it seems that the nation-state has imparted special symbolic and practical meaning to the lives of individuals and groups, who, in turn, have become involved in a constant negotiation with their homeland over crucial emotional and social attitudes, such as shared destiny, loyalty, and solidarity (Hazan and Monterescu, 2011).

Despite their professional attitude towards mental vulnerability, the Israeli experts and therapists dealing with trauma were clearly acting in strong reference to this collectivist world view. Core national values, as well as the Zionist narrative of building a Jewish state on the land of Israel, have shaped the professional management of trauma by the mental health experts, as well as the resistance expressed to them by the diverse local populations. From the outset, the experts focused their attention on an initial formulation of traumatic injury rooted in the political equation of "we the Jews" versus "them the Arabs." This therapeutic stance assumed a kind of symbiosis, real or imaginary, between the individual and the national collective, and both NATAL and ITC justified their exclusive dealing with trauma and PTSD in the context of the Arab–Israeli conflict on this basis. Their deliberate abstention from dealing with other kinds of trauma, such as traffic accidents or sexual abuse, was that they differed fundamentally from security-based trauma. The mental injury to the individual from security-based trauma, they explained, was in many ways an injury due to an event perpetrated against him or her as an integral part of the collective. Therefore, the individual must be acknowledged and treated and, as such, the collective would be acknowledged and treated.

This link between trauma management and collectivist moral sentiment is further accentuated in light of the fact that it touches upon one of Israel's underlying emotional crossroads: victimization versus heroism (Bilu and Witztum, 2000; Kidron, 2004; Kimmerling, 1993). The emergence of the State of Israel out of the Holocaust interwove Jewish victimization into the Zionist narrative. However, at the same time, it marked Israel's birth as a sovereign entity with the capacity for endurance and fighting. Almost unnoticed, this historic tension between the "old Jew," identified as passive and weak of body, and the "new Jew," characterized by a stalwart physique and fighting strength, migrated to the contemporary professional approach to mental vulnerability. On the one hand, the mental condition of trauma resulting from the Arab–Israeli conflict became highly recognized by the Israeli public. This recognition opened a new way for Israelis to define their mental state in relation to the political conflict as one of traumatic or post-traumatic suffering. This new development sketched a current interface between daily life in contemporary Israel and the traditional, well-known victimized stance, the one identified with passivity, dysfunction, and dissolution.

On the other hand, the expansion of the professional management of trauma from the clinical label associated with the individual (through terms such as "PTSD" or "secondary trauma") to programs aimed to fortifying entire communities (through terms such as "at-risk groups," "resilience," and "immunization") made it possible to sketch an additional, alternative interface. This interface took the opposite emotional and social stance – that of heroism. Just as trauma and PTSD became an elegant, contemporary improvement on victimization, so too resilience became an elegant, contemporary improvement on patriotism, strength, and the capacity to endure.

Thus, the professional approach of NATAL and ITC worked in two directions simultaneously. The first direction was thrust into motion by the medicalized model of trauma backed by the individualistic orientation. This dynamic had the ability to "suspend," at least for a limited period of time, political controversies and to create some kind of intended "blindness" to the internal stratification between various ethnic populations in Israel. The second direction grew out of the increased legitimacy of the terms "trauma" and "PTSD" and out of the powerful ties between those definitions and some core national values. Both NGOs were driven by the Zionist narrative of Israel, which in many ways shaped the moral boundaries of their professional attitude and limited their scope of activity primarily to the Jewish residents of Israel.

This blend of the individualistic and collectivistic systems of giving meaning to the professional management of trauma in Israel led to the orchestration of a new therapeutic contract. Rather than the classic, individualistic mode of therapist versus patient interacting with each other within the secret confines of the clinic, a new intermeshed individual-collective mode of dialogue was gradually constructed. This new contract was based on mental health experts with diverse professional training (psychiatrists, clinical psychologists, psychotherapists, social workers, and educational consultants) engaging with various groups of patients, semi-patients, and non-patients and their mental vulnerabilities of differing degrees inside but mostly outside the clinic. Between those aid providers and aid receivers the clinical definitions of trauma and PTSD had been perceived as fundamentally tied to the individual, aimed at the "universal man" and "universal woman" (Malkki, 1996), thus independently applied. Nevertheless, addressing security-based mental vulnerability turned out to be effective in eliciting all those communal experiences of socio-economic inequality and class and ethnic differences, typically silenced or pushed aside when the focus was on the individual. Therefore, the professional engagement with trauma and PTSD changed from strictly dealing with psychiatric definitions and mental symptoms to a new contract that allowed the expression and sharing of diverse, subjective interpretations of national belonging. Accordingly, it at least has the potential to bridge the gap between diverse populations of Israeli residents, Jewish and non-Jewish, and Jews from different ethnic, religious, and socio-economic backgrounds, each of them with their own historical and contemporary experiences of everyday life in Israel under the current security circumstances.

Within this new therapeutic contract, the mental health experts from NATAL and ITC have been applying three practices in order to stabilize their position between the clinical and political dimensions, and they have done so using both an individual focus and the ongoing presence of collectivistic values. First, there was a blurring of the "political" for the sake of emphasizing the "clinical." Second, there was a blurring of the "clinical" for the sake of emphasizing the "political." Lastly, there was a mix, a blurring of the "political" for the sake of emphasizing the "clinical," and then a connection back to the "political" once again.

The first practice, and perhaps the most surprising, was based on the new professional attention being given to the political dimension of mental vulnerability in the current context of the conflict. This practice was applied, for example, in the town of Sderot (chapter 7). In this context, the NGOs identified the entire community as a site for intervention under the Building Resilience Program, while taking into account the particular cultural background of the local population and the socio-economic circumstances of their daily lives. In addition, as a part of the intervention program, repeated associations between the clinical label of trauma and social labelling became evident.

The second practice on which the new therapeutic contract was based went in the opposite direction, namely, by pushing aside or blurring the political dimension for the sake of emphasizing the clinical-individual one. An example was the case regarding the Jewish evacuees from the Gaza Strip and the West Bank (chapter 1). In the face of a fierce political dispute, the Israeli therapists made intensive efforts to situate the evacuees in an apolitical position of "those in need" beyond the public debate. Struggling for empirical evidence of the evacuees' mental distress, ITC council members tried to legitimize the allocation of financial and organizational resources for aid intervention.

The third and last practice the mental health experts applied was to erase the political dimension and then retag it. The situation of the Palestinian citizens of Israel in the wake of the Second Lebanon War (chapter 1) demonstrates this practice. Their intensive exposure to rocket fire led to the establishment of a professional niche for this specific audience (the "Arab target group"). Subsequently, there was renewed political debate, but their weakened civil position did not afford them full organizational recognition. Another group in a vulnerable civic position in Israeli society, the bereaved Druze parents from Dalyat el-Carmel (chapter 6), also typifies the third practice. At first, the therapists referred to the complex political context in which the bereavement of this ethno-national minority developed. However, afterwards the therapists glossed over it when they adhered to the neutral clinical definition as the point of departure for receiving aid ("traumatic grief").

Treading cautiously around the sensitive clinical and political domains is far from an expected process in the mental health community in Israel. As described in earlier studies, the existing tendency among Israeli therapists has been to huddle within the boundaries of the clinic and keep their distance from anything perceived as "political" (Berman, 2003). In contrast, the therapists from NATAL and ITC sought to create new ways of involvement. They took into consideration all the highly charged points of contact between the clinical and the political, and between the therapeutic and the national. Unlike their colleagues in the past, they were not doing so from inside state institutions (Bilu and Witztum, 2000). They were also not crudely wielding therapeutic language for the sake of dealing with issues of ethnic and class inequality (Mizrachi, 2004). Instead, they were acting from the more liberal-individualistic stance of civil society, while cautiously, and at times creatively, applying the national-collectivistic world view.

Orchestrating a new therapeutic contract based on creative navigation between the clinical and political domains crossed over from the therapists to the patients. The participants' responses to the experts' offers and messages during the therapeutic interventions, and to their mental vulnerability in face of security threats, uncovered a world of meaning often awarded precedence to components of group identity, such as religion, ethnicity, gender, and class, over any universal or liberal-individual concepts. The various groups of participants often perceived the individualistic message underlying the therapeutic work as a threat to their traditional group identities. This way of interpretation was evident, for example, among the repatriated Jewish POWs (chapter 4), the bereaved Druze parents of Dalyat el-Carmel, the Bedouin social workers, and the children of Kibbutz Zikkim (chapter 6). Against the therapeutic message to frame their experiences as individual ones, then to label them under terms such as trauma or post-trauma, their social codes emerged. Political positions and experiences of inequalities that strongly shaped their daily life rose to the surface and exposed the boundary lines and power dynamics that their therapists tended to push aside, maybe a bit too far. How far away is the southern town of Sderot from Israel's strong Ashkenazi centre? Can the local meaning of the masculine identity serve as an effective framework to cope with the mental difficulties of military service and captivity? And, if not, to what extent can treatment be used without completely negating it? How differently does a Bedouin social worker go about calming an anxious patient than does a Jewish clinical psychologist? To what extent and until when should a woman limit and narrow her own world in order to support her spouse who suffers from attacks of rage after collecting body parts at the site of a terror attack? How can she love and feel loved in the face of the withdrawal and avoidance that now characterize his behaviour? How different is the Israeli soldier who attacks a Palestinian civilian from that civilian himself, if both of them are close to the clinical nucleus of PTSD? Is it legitimate to talk about trauma in the plural voice, as did Shai, the firefighter who evacuated the wounded from the Park Hotel on Passover Eve? Or is it more accurate to do so in the singular voice, as the marketing adviser asked him to do? Can the emotional alliance of bereavement between Druze and Jewish parents reduce the ethno-national distance between them? Or should there even be an attempt made to unite these two groups given their religious and historical differences?

Sometimes these questions cropped up cautiously, through a hint or passing allusion, for example, in the clinical treatment of the soldier who was considering filing a lawsuit against the Ministry of Defense. Nonetheless, similar questions were also expressed loudly during the sessions of the support group for women who were married to men diagnosed with PTSD, when their very intimate stories evoked strong criticism against state agencies such as the Ministry of Defense and the National Insurance Institute. Sometimes these questions seemed to flood the room, turning the tables on the therapists and presenting them with an alternative agenda. Instances of this alternative agenda included the workshop for the residents of the Neve Eshkol neighbourhood in Sderot, the end of the study day for bereaved parents in Dalyat el-Carmel, and the play staged by the children of Kibbutz Zikkim in the south. All in all, whether in passing allusion or in a flood, whether cautiously or bluntly, dealing with these questions exposed the nature of the new therapeutic contract that evolved around the mental condition of trauma.

The right to conclude is reserved for the people who stood at the centre of the study: aid providers and aid receivers. The ethnographic journey regarding trauma management – which rests upon a variety of couches, chairs, benches, and mats – ended at Tel Aviv University on a

Saturday evening, 12 July 2008. To mark the second anniversary of the abduction of IDF soldiers along the Lebanese border, in a festive but tense atmosphere, a select audience watched *My First War*, a movie by Yariv Moser. In the movie, Moser recounted his experiences from the long days of the war and his encounters with soldiers and journalists during its course. At the end of the screening, Moser invited the participants of the movie to the stage, as well as Dr. Itamar Barnea, NATAL's chief psychologist. Barnea opened the conversation:

> DR. BARNEA: You are a group of charming people, entirely random, who represent each and every one of us in this country. The movie connected each of us to the great pain of the outcomes of war and the continuing madness from one war to another in this country. I would like to thank you.
>
> YARIV MOSER (THE DIRECTOR): [In light of the mental hardships described by the participants in the movie], is it recommended to do reserve duty? To go to the next war?
>
> DR. BARNEA (slightly embarrassed): May there not be a next war ... Each one in keeping with his own ability and his own way of coping. I, as a psychologist, won't recommend participating or not participating in the next war.
>
> MOSER (to one of the movie's participants, Ido Meller): Will you go to the next war?
>
> IDO MELLER: It's not that I have a choice ... As I also said to my parents, in this war I didn't get killed. It'll probably happen next time.
>
> DR. BARNEA (looking at Meller): Everyone is looking to find themselves, because that's where they feel human ... And that, ultimately, is what everyone wants to feel. (12 July 2008, Field Notes)

Afterwards, Barnea said that he had given Meller his calling card. Maybe he will come, so they can talk.

References

Abramowitz, Sharon Alane. 2010. "Trauma and Humanitarian Translation in Liberia: The Tale of Open Mole." *Culture, Medicine and Psychiatry* 34 (2): 353–79. http://dx.doi.org/10.1007/s11013-010-9172-0

Abu-Rabia-Queder, Sarab. 2008. *Excluded and Loved: Educated Bedouin Women's Life Stories*. Jerusalem: Eshkolot and Magnes, The Hebrew University of Jerusalem Press. (in Hebrew).

Adams, Vincanne, Taslim Van Hattum, and Diana English. 2009. "Chronic Disaster Syndrome: Displacement, Disaster Capitalism and the Eviction of the Poor from New Orleans." *American Ethnologist* 36 (4): 615–36. http://dx.doi.org/10.1111/j.1548-1425.2009.01199.x

Alexander, Jeffrey C. 2004. "Toward a Theory of Cultural Trauma." In *Cultural Trauma and Collective Identity*, edited by Jeffrey C. Alexander, Ron Eyerman, Bernhard Giesen, Neil J. Smelser, and Piotr Sztompka, 1–30. Berkeley: University of California Press. http://dx.doi.org/10.1525/california/9780520235946.003.0001

Appadurai, Arjun. 1996. *Modernity at Large: Cultural Dimensions of Globalization*. Minneapolis: University of Minnesota Press.

Beck, Ulrich. 2006. *The Cosmopolitan Vision*. Cambridge: Polity Press.

Berman, Emanual. 2003. "Israeli Psychotherapists and the Israeli-Palestinian Conflict." *Psychotherapy and Politics International* 1 (1): 1–16. http://dx.doi.org/10.1002/ppi.47

Bilu, Yoram, and Eliezer Witztum. 2000. "War-Related Loss and Suffering in Israeli Society: An Historical Perspective." *Israel Studies* 5 (2): 1–31. http://dx.doi.org/10.2979/ISR.2000.5.2.1

Bleich, Avraham, Marc Gelkopf, and Zahava Solomon. 2003. "Exposure to Terrorism, Stress-Related Mental Health Symptoms and Coping Behaviors among a Nationality Representative Sample in Israel." *Journal of the*

American Medical Association 290 (5): 612–20. http://dx.doi.org/10.1001/
jama.290.5.612

Bob, Clifford. 2002. "Merchants of Morality." *Foreign Policy* 129 (Mar–Apr):
36–45. http://dx.doi.org/10.2307/3183388

Boltanski, Luc. 1999. *Distant Suffering: Morality, Media and Politics*. Cambridge:
Cambridge University Press.

Bornstein, Erica. 2009. "The Impulse of Philanthropy." *Cultural Anthropology*
24 (4): 622–51. http://dx.doi.org/10.1111/j.1548-1360.2009.01042.x

Bracken, Patrick J. 1998. "Hidden Agendas: Deconstructing Post Traumatic
Stress Disorder." In *Rethinking the Trauma of War*, edited by Patrick J.
Bracken and Celia Petty, 38–59. New York: Free Association Books.

Breslau, Joshua. 2004. "Introduction: Cultures of Trauma: Anthropology
Views of Posttraumatic Stress Disorder in International Health." *Culture,
Medicine and Psychiatry* 28 (2): 113–26. http://dx.doi.org/10.1023/
B:MEDI.0000034421.07612.c8

Brunner, Jose. 2006. "The Unending Story: Trauma and Ideology in the
Shadow of Al-Aqsa Intifada." *Theory and Criticism* 28: 231–9. (in Hebrew)

Danieli, Yael, Danny Brom, and Joe Sills, eds. 2005. *The Trauma of
Terrorism: Sharing Knowledge and Sharing Care, An International Handbook*.
Binghampton, UK: The Haworth Press.

Dekel, Rachel, Hadas Goldblatt, Michal Keidar, Zahava Solomon, and
Michael Polliack. 2005. "Being a Wife of a Veteran with Posttraumatic Stress
Disorder." *Family Relations* 54 (1): 24–36. http://dx.doi.org/10.1111/j.0197-
6664.2005.00003.x

Dickson-Go'mez, Julia. 2002. "The Sound of Barking Dogs: Violence and
Terror among Salvadoran Families in the Postwar." *Medical Anthropology
Quarterly* 16 (4): 348–415.

Dwyer, Leslie, and Degung Santikarma. 2007. "Posttraumatic Politics:
Violence, Memory, and Biomedical Discourse in Bali." In *Understanding
Trauma: Integrating Biological, Clinical, and Cultural Perspectives*, edited
by Lourence J. Kirmayer, Robert Lemelson, and Mark Barad, 403–32.
Cambridge: Cambridge University Press. http://dx.doi.org/10.1017/
CBO9780511500008.025

Egeland, Byron, Elizabeth Carlson, and Alan L. Sroufe. 1993. "Resilience as
Process." *Development and Psychopathology* 5 (4): 517–28. http://dx.doi.org/
10.1017/S0954579400006131

Elisha, Omri. 2008. "Moral Ambitions of Grace: The Paradox of Compassion
and Accountability in Evangelical Faith-Based Activism." *Cultural
Anthropology* 23 (1): 154–89. http://dx.doi.org/10.1111/j.1548-1360.
2008.00006.x

Fassin, Didier. 2008. "The Humanitarian Politics of Testimony: Subjectification through Trauma in the Israeli-Palestinian Conflict." *Cultural Anthropology* 23 (3): 531–58. http://dx.doi.org/10.1111/j.1548-1360.2008.00017.x

Fassin, Didier, and Richard Rechtman. 2009. *The Empire of Trauma: An Inquiry into the Condition of Victimhood*. Princeton, NJ: Princeton University Press.

Finley, Erin. 2015. "The Chaplain Turns to God: Negotiating Posttraumatic Stress Disorder in the American Military." In *Genocide and Mass Violence: Memory, Symptoms, and Recovery*, edited by Devon E. Hinton and Alexander L. Hinton, 263–79. Cambridge: Cambridge University Press.

Foucault, Michel. 1973. *The Birth of the Clinic: An Archaeology of Medical Perception*. New York: Vintage Books.

Furedi, Frank. 2004. *Therapy Culture: Cultivating Vulnerability in an Uncertain Age*. New York: Routledge.

Gaines, Atwood D. 1992. "From DSM-I to III-R; Voices of Self, Mastery, and the Other: A Cultural Constructivist Reading of U.S. Psychiatry Classification." *Social Science & Medicine* 35 (1): 3–24. http://dx.doi.org/10.1016/0277-9536(92)90115-7

Gal, Reuven. 1990. "Psychological and Moral Aspects of IDF's Soldiers Coping with the Intifada." In *The Seventh War: The Effects of the Intifada on Israeli Society*, edited by Reuven Gal, 149–55. Tel Aviv: HaKibbutz HaMeuchad. (in Hebrew)

Gieryn, Thomas F. 1999. *Cultural Boundaries of Science: Credibility on the Line*. Chicago: University of Chicago Press.

Good, Byron. 1994. *Medicine, Rationality, and Experience: An Anthropological Perspective*. Cambridge: Cambridge University Press.

Hacking, Ian. 1986. "Making Up People." In *Reconstructing Individualism: Autonomy, Individuality, and the Self in Western Thought*, edited by Thomas C. Heller, Morton Sosna, and David E. Wellbery, 222–36. Palo Alto, CA: Stanford University Press.

– 1996. "Memory Science, Memory Politics." In *Tense Past: Cultural Essays in Trauma and Memory*, edited by Paul Antze and Michael Lambek, 67–87. New York: Routledge.

Halbwachs, Maurice. 1992. *On Collective Memory*. Chicago: University of Chicago Press.

Han, Clara. 2004. "The Work of Indebtedness: The Traumatic Present of Late Capitalist Chile." *Culture, Medicine and Psychiatry* 28 (2): 169–87. http://dx.doi.org/10.1023/B:MEDI.0000034409.70790.66

Hazan, Haim, and Daniel Monterescu. 2011. *A Town at Sundown: Aging Nationalism in Jaffa*. Jerusalem: Van Leer Jerusalem Institute and HaKibbutz Hameuchad. (in Hebrew)

Herman, Judith Lewis. 1992. *Trauma and Recovery*. New York: Basic Books.

Herzog, Hanna. 1999. *Gendering Politics: Women in Israel*. Ann Arbor: University of Michigan Press.

Illouz, Eva. 2008. *Saving the Modern Soul: Therapy, Emotions, and the Culture of Self-Help*. Berkeley: University of California Press.

James, Erica Caple. 2004. "The Political Economy of 'Trauma' in Haiti in the Democratic Era of Insecurity." *Culture, Medicine and Psychiatry* 28 (2): 127–49. http://dx.doi.org/10.1023/B:MEDI.0000034407.39471.d4

Jordan, B. Kathleen, Charles R. Marmar, John A. Fairbank, William E. Schlenger, Richard A. Kulka, Richard L. Hough, and Daniel S. Weiss. 1992. "Problems in Families of Male Vietnam Veterans with Posttraumatic Stress Disorder." *Journal of Consulting and Clinical Psychology* 60 (6): 916–26.

Kidron, Carol A. 2004. "Surviving a Distant Past: Study of the Cultural Construction of Trauma Descendant Identity." *Ethos* 31 (14): 513–44.

Kimmerling, Baruch. 1993. "Patterns of Militarism in Israel." *Archives Européennes de Sociologie* 34 (2): 1–28.

Kirmayer, Laurence J. 2015. "Commentary: Wrestling With the Angles of History: Memory, Symptoms, and Intervention." In *Genocide and Mass Violence: Memory, Symptoms, and Recovery*, edited by Devon E. Hinton and Alexander L. Hinton, 388–420. Cambridge: Cambridge University Press.

Kleinman, Arthur. 1995. *Writing at the Margin: Discourse between Anthropology and Medicine*. Berkeley: University of California Press.

Knafo, Daniella, ed. 2004. *Living with Terror, Working with Trauma: A Clinician's Handbook*. Lanham: Rowman and Littlefield.

Kobasa, Suzanne C. 1982. "The Hardy Personality: Toward a Social Psychology of Stress and Health." In *Social Psychology of Health and Illness*, edited by Glenn S. Sander and Jerry Suls, 3–32. Hillsdale, NJ: Erlbaum Publishers.

Kutchins, Herb, and Stuart A. Kirk. 1997. *Making Us Crazy*. New York: The Free Press.

Lieblich, A. 1978. *The Soldiers on Jerusalem Beach*. New York: Random House.

Lomsky-Feder, Edna. 2004. "Life Stories, War, and Veterans: On the Social Distribution of Memories." *Ethos* 32 (1): 82–109. http://dx.doi.org/10.1525/eth.2004.32.1.82

Lomsky-Feder, Edna, and Eyal Ben-Ari. 2011. "Trauma, Therapy and Responsibility: Psychology and War in Contemporary Israel." In *The Practice of War: Production, Reproduction and Communication of Armed Violence*, edited by Aparna Rao, Michael Bolling, and Monika Bock, 111–31. New York: Berghahn Books.

Luhrmann, Tanya M. 2010. "Review of *The Empire of Trauma: An Inquiry into the Condition of Victimhood*, by Didier Fassin and Richard Rechtman. Translated by Rachel Gomme." *American Journal of Psychiatry* 167 (6): 722. http://ajp.psychiatryonline.org/doi/abs/10.1176/appi.ajp.2010.09121821

Malkki, Lisa H. 1996. "Speechless Emissaries: Refugees, Humanitarianism and Dehistoricization." *Cultural Anthropology* 11 (3): 377–404. http://dx.doi .org/10.1525/can.1996.11.3.02a00050

Milgram, Noach. 1994. "Psychological Study in Israel During the Gulf War." *Psychology* 4 (1–2): 7–17. (in Hebrew)

Milliken, C.S., J.L. Auchterlonie, and C.W. Hoge. 2007. "Longitudinal Assessment of Mental Health Problems among Active and Reserve Component Soldiers Returning from the Iraq War." *Journal of the American Medical Association* 298 (18): 2141–48. http://dx.doi.org/10.1001/jama.298.18.2141

Mizrachi, Nissim. 2004. "From Badness to Sickness: The Role of Ethnopsychology in Shaping Ethnic Hierarchies in Israel." *Social Identities* 10 (2): 219–43. http://dx.doi.org/10.1080/1350463042000227362

Monson, Candice M., Casey T. Taft, and Steffany J. Fredman. 2009. "Military-Related PTSD and Intimate Relationships: From Description to Theory-Driven Research and Intervention Development." *Clinical Psychology Review* 29 (8): 707–14. http://dx.doi.org/10.1016/j.cpr.2009.09.002

Moore, Dahlia. 2012. *Two Steps Forward, One Step Back: Changing Women, Changing Society*. Boston: Academic Studies Press.

Murphy, Raymond. 1988. *Social Closure: The Theory of Monopolization and Exclusion*. New York: Oxford University Press.

Neriya, Yuval. 1994. *Life in the Shadow of War: Psychological Aspects*. Jerusalem: Davis Institute for International Relationships, the Hebrew University of Jerusalem. (in Hebrew)

Ortner, Sherrey B. 1973. "On Key Symbols." *American Anthropologist* 75 (5): 1338–46. http://dx.doi.org/10.1525/aa.1973.75.5.02a00100

Parson, Nia. 2010. "Transformative Ties: Gendered Violence, Forms of Recovery and Shifting Subjectivity in Chile." *Medical Anthropology Quarterly* 24 (1): 64–84. http://dx.doi.org/10.1111/j.1548-1387.2010.01085.x

Plotkin-Amrami, Galia. 2013. "Between National Ideology and Western Therapy: On the Emergence of a New 'Culture of Trauma' Following the 2005 Forced Evacuation of Jewish Israeli Settlers." *Transcult Psychiatry* (50) 1: 47–67. http://dx.doi.org/10.1177/1363461513479760

Pupavac, Venessa. 2001. "Therapeutic Governance: Psycho-Social Intervention and Trauma Risk Management." *Disaster* 25 (4): 358–72. http://dx.doi .org/10.1111/1467-7717.00184

Rabinowitz, Dan. 2001. "The Palestinian Citizens of Israel, the Concept of Trapped Minority and the Discourse of Transnationalism." *Ethnic and Racial Studies* 24 (1): 64–85. http://dx.doi.org/10.1080/014198701750052505

Redfield, Peter. 2006. "A Less Modest Witness: Collective Advocacy and Motivated Truth in a Medical Humanitarian Movement." *American Ethnologist* 33 (1): 3–26. http://dx.doi.org/10.1525/ae.2006.33.1.3

Rhodes, R.A.W. 1996. "The New Governance: Governing Without Government." *Political Studies* 44 (4): 652–67. http://dx.doi.org/10.1111/j.1467-9248.1996.tb01747.x

Richardson, Glenn E. 2002. "The Metatheory of Resilience and Resiliency." *Journal of Clinical Psychology* 58 (3): 307–21. http://dx.doi.org/10.1002/jclp.10020

Rose, Nikolas. 1998. *Inventing Ourselves: Psychology, Power and Personhood.* Cambridge: Cambridge University Press.

Sachs, Dalia, Amlia Sa'ar, and Sarai Aharoni. 2007. "'How Can I Feel for Others when I Myself Am Beaten?' The Impact of the Armed Conflict on Women in Israel." *Sex Roles* 57 (7–8): 593–606. http://dx.doi.org/10.1007/s11199-007-9222-4

Sayers, Steven L., Victoria A. Farrow, Jennifer Ross, and David W. Oslin. 2009. "Family Problems among Recently Returned Military Veterans Referred for a Mental Health Evaluation." *Journal of Clinical Psychiatry* 70 (2): 163–70. http://dx.doi.org/10.4088/JCP.07m03863.

Shafir, Gershon, and Yoav Peled. 2002. *Being Israeli: The Dynamics of Multiple Citizenship.* Cambridge: Cambridge University Press. http://dx.doi.org/10.1017/CBO9781139164641

Shamgar-Handelman, Lea. 1986. *Israeli War Widows: Beyond the Glory of Heroism.* South Hadley, MA: Bergin and Garvey Publishers.

Shamir, Ronen. 2008. "The Age of Responsibilization: On Market-Embedded Morality." *Economy and Society* 37 (1): 1–19. http://dx.doi.org/10.1080/03085140701760833

Shokeid, Moshe. 1997. "Negotiating Multiple Viewpoints: The Cook, the Native, the Publishers and the Ethnographic Text." *Current Anthropology* 38 (4): 631–45. http://dx.doi.org/10.1086/204649

Silber, Ilana. 2008. "A New Era for Philanthropists? The Case of Israel." *Civic Society and Third Sector in Israel* 2 (1): 9–32. (in Hebrew)

Silver, Roxane, Cohen, Alison Holman, Daniel N. Mcintosh, Michael Poulin, and Virginia Gil-Rivas. 2002. "Nationwide Longitudinal Study of Psychological Responses to September 11." *Journal of the American Medical Association* 288 (10): 1235–44. http://dx.doi.org/10.1001/jama.288.10.1235

Solomon, Zehava. 1993. *Combat Stress Reaction: The Enduring Toll of War*. New York: Plenum Press.

Solomon, Zahava, Rachel Dekel, and Gadi Zerach. 2008. "The Relationships between Posttraumatic Stress Symptoms Clusters and Marital Intimacy among War Veterans." *Journal of Family Psychology* 22 (5): 659–66. http://dx.doi.org/10.1037/a0013596

Somer, Eli, and Avraham Bleich, eds. 2005. *Mental Health in Terror's Shadow: The Israeli Experience*. Tel-Aviv, Ramot: Tel-Aviv University Press. (in Hebrew)

Trani, Jean-François, and Parul Bakshi. 2013. "Vulnerability and Mental Health in Afghanistan: Looking Beyond War Exposure." *Transcultural Psychiatry* 50 (1): 108–39. http://dx.doi.org/10.1177/1363461512475025

Tzfadia, Erez, and Oren Yiftachel. 2004. "Between Urban and National: Political Mobilization among Mizrahim in Israel's 'Developments Towns.'" *Cities* 21 (1): 41–55. http://dx.doi.org/10.1016/j.cities.2003.10.006

Warner, Faith R. 2007. "Social Support and Distress among Q'eqchi' Refugee Women in Maya Tecu'n, Mexico." *Medical Anthropology Quarterly* 21 (2): 193–217. http://dx.doi.org/10.1525/maq.2007.21.2.193

Wilson, R.A. 2000. "Reconciliation and Revenge in Post–Apartheid South Africa." *Current Anthropology* 41 (1): 75–98. http://dx.doi.org/10.1086/300104

Ya'ar, Ephraim, and Efrat Peleg. 2007. *Patriotism and National Resilience in Israel: The Survey of Patriotism 2007*. Herzelia: The Institute of Policy and Strategy. (in Hebrew)

Young, Allan. 1995. *The Harmony of Illusion: Inventing Post-Traumatic Stress Disorder*. Princeton, NJ: Princeton University Press.

– 2002. "The Self-Traumatized Perpetrator as a 'Transient Mental Illness.'" *L'Évolution Psychiatrique* 67 (4): 630–50. http://dx.doi.org/10.1016/S0014-3855(02)00162-7

– 2007. "Posttraumatic Stress Disorder of the Virtual Kind: Trauma and Resilience in Post 9/11 America." In *Trauma and Memory: Reading, Healing and Making Law*, edited by Austin Sarat, Nadav Davidovich, and Michal Alberstein, 21–48. Palo Alto, CA: Stanford University Press.

Zarowsky, Christina. 2004. "Writing Trauma: Emotion, Ethnography and the Politics of Suffering among Somali Returnees in Ethiopia." *Culture, Medicine and Psychiatry* 28 (2): 189–209. http://dx.doi.org/10.1023/B:MEDI.0000034410.08428.29

Index